Living Well Without a Gallbladder
A Guide to Postcholecystectomy Syndrome

By Brooke Keefer

Copyright and Disclaimer

Dedication and Acknowledgments

This book is dedicated to postcholecystectomy patients, their families, caregivers, and friends. May this book help bring wellness back into your lives. This is as much your book as it is mine.

I would like to pay special thanks to my family, especially my mother (Linda Valerino), father (Donald Valerino), stepmother (Janice Valerino), stepfather (John Saladin), and children (Alex, Schyler, and William).

Thank you to my friends who have gotten me through the worst of times and never gave up faith in me. Special thanks to all the compassionate, supportive doctors out there.

Table of Contents

Introduction

In 1998, I was told by my doctor that I needed to have my gallbladder removed after I'd been experiencing nausea and pressure under my sternum for several weeks. My symptoms weren't life-threatening or disabling, but were uncomfortable and interfering with my ability to work and parent my children.

An ultrasound revealed that my gallbladder was full of gallstones. At the time, I had no idea what a gallstone was or the gallbladder's purpose. I was 29 years old and couldn't believe this was happening to me. The only people I knew who had gallbladder issues were people over 40.

I couldn't help but wonder how I developed gallstones. Possibly it was from drinking too much bourbon (I promptly quit drinking around the time of this diagnosis). Maybe it was all the cheese and other fatty foods I ate. I was only 120 pounds. Therefore, it couldn't have been my weight.

Regardless of the reason I had gallstones, I was relieved when the doctor told me the fix would be easy—a simple outpatient surgery. He told me I really didn't need my gallbladder, that it was as useful as the appendix. Since I did not like feeling crappy day in and day out, I jumped at the opportunity to have this "useless" organ removed.

Within a few weeks of my diagnosis, I had my gallbladder removed laparoscopically, a minimally invasive procedure known as cholecystectomy (pronounced koh-luh-si-stek-tuh-mee). The surgery was straightforward without complications. I was in and out of the hospital like going through a drive-thru at a fast food restaurant. The recovery was a breeze as well and the minute scars made it appear as though I never had an organ removed.

I experienced minimal post-surgical pain and felt better within a few days. Initially, I was pleased with the surgery. However, two weeks later, I did not feel the same sentiment. I developed a stabbing pain in my right side, under my rib cage that radiated up my back and shoulder. It felt like a hot poker was stabbing and twisting inside me and was debilitating. I also had loose stools, which was odd because I was almost always constipated.

My primary care doctor suspected the diarrhea was caused by excess bile or bile acid malabsorption and prescribed a bile acid sequestrant. Although the medication resolved my diarrhea, my doctor did not have an explanation or solution for the pain I was experiencing.

To pinpoint the cause of the pain, I was referred to a gastroenterologist who ordered an endoscopy and barium enema. The results were normal, other than the endoscopy showed I had bile refluxing into my stomach. Bile reflux can be painful, but typically it feels more like acid reflux. It can also cause nausea and a burning sensation in the esophagus.

Unable to find an organic cause for the pain, the gastroenterologist diagnosed me with Irritable Bowel Syndrome (IBS) and prescribed an antispasmodic medication, which did nothing for the pain. I began to notice the pain was worse after eating, if I hadn't eaten in a while, and during times of stress. As days went on, the pain worsened and completely interfered with my day to day life.

Left with no medication, no concrete diagnosis or any solution for my pain, I learned natural ways to control it and went on with my life. I accepted the pain was from IBS, but wasn't entirely convinced since the pain was too high to be bowel-related. I lived a normal healthy life thereafter, utilizing deep breathing, yoga, dietary modifications, and medication to keep the pain in check. In time, my bile acid diarrhea subsided, and I developed the opposite problem—constipation, probably from lack of bile postcholecystectomy.

In 2011, while pregnant with my third son, the right-side pain magically disappeared for the first time in 13 years. I delivered a healthy child and seemed to be doing well digestive-wise. Three months post-partum I suddenly developed nasty symptoms. I had nausea around the clock which led to constant vomiting, the inability to keep weight on, and had severe pain under my sternum.

I was very ill, requiring several hospitalizations. Most of my local doctors were convinced my symptoms were psychological in nature since my bloodwork and scans were normal. My family and I knew differently and were elated when a local surgeon I consulted suggested I might have sphincter of Oddi dysfunction (SOD). I say elated because not knowing what was wrong with me was about as bad as the symptoms themselves.

I researched SOD thoroughly and found it was most common in women who had their gallbladders removed. All the symptoms matched mine. I learned through support groups and the Internet there was a doctor at the University of Minnesota who was an SOD specialist. Not getting anywhere with my local doctors, it became my mission to travel across the country to see this doctor.

By the time I saw the Minnesota doctor, I had endured eight months of malnutrition, significant weight loss, pain, scrutiny by doctors, and multiple emergency room and hospital visits. During the first consult with this doctor, he told me he thought I had SOD but wanted me to gain weight prior to performing the diagnostic procedure and treatment. He was compassionate and validated my symptoms, something that was missing from my local gastroenterologist.

I returned home and had a feeding tube surgically placed in my abdomen. I didn't have the greatest experience with the feeding tube, but it did enable me to gain enough weight to return to Minnesota for the SOD procedure, an ERCP with manometry and sphincterotomy (cutting of the biliary and pancreatic sphincters), which was the gold standard for diagnosing SOD. Sure enough, after a year of normal test results, I was diagnosed with SOD. The ERCP with manometry measured the pressures of my biliary and pancreatic sphincters. My pressures were three to four times higher than the norm.

Sadly, I developed acute pancreatitis and sepsis from the procedure. The doctor told my mom, while I was lying in bed on a ventilator, I would likely die. Obviously, I didn't die. After a one-week stay in the intensive care unit of the hospital, I recovered and flew home to New York. The procedure helped my symptoms for a few weeks. However, they eventually returned. A local surgeon recommended I have major abdominal surgery, a transduodenal sphincteroplasty, where the biliary and pancreatic sphincters would be sewn permanently open.

I elected to have the surgery, but ended up with sepsis again and was essentially poisoned by Levaquin, a fluoroquinolone antibiotic, they administered. This resulted in tendinopathy, neuropathy, and central nervous system damage. I am still recovering from that but at least the sphincteroplasty resolved my SOD issues. Now I have occasional bile reflux and bowel issues but manage them well. I also have chronic pancreatitis, which could have been triggered by the sphincteroplasty or the acute pancreatitis episode, or really anything as its origin is unknown.

During my illness, I vowed that when I felt better, I would dedicate my life to educating people about SOD and postcholecystectomy syndrome. In July 2016, after several years of research and interviewing patients, I published *The Sphincter of Oddi Dysfunction Survival Guide.* As of this writing, it is the only book written about SOD by an SOD patient.

It only made sense for me to continue writing about postcholecystectomy issues. Though many people feel great and "normal" years after cholecystectomy, the research and my experience show there is still a percentage of patients who do not fare well without a gallbladder. To make matters worse, there are doctors who don't believe in postcholecystectomy syndrome.

Prior to writing *Living Well Without a Gallbladder*, I searched various online bookstores for post-gallbladder and postcholecystectomy topics. Overall, not much surfaced about postcholecystectomy syndrome anywhere on the Internet, aside from a few dedicated sites, forums, and people selling miracle cures. Clearly there was a need for a book to be written for postcholecystectomy patients experiencing complications and symptoms following their surgery.

Though I am not a doctor, and none of the information contained in this book is to be used as medical advice, I have the advantage of writing about postcholecystectomy syndrome from the patient's perspective. In no way am I intending to diagnose or treat any person's condition. That is the job of a doctor or other healthcare professional.

Use this book as a tool and not a prescription. Always consult with your doctors about introducing a treatment or removing a treatment. Do not self-medicate, even with natural remedies like supplements and herbs. They can be contraindicated for your condition or interact with medications you are taking.

Remember as you read this book that my story is a worst-case scenario of sorts. Do not think everything I experienced will happen to you. Also, do not jump to the conclusion that every postcholecystectomy condition described herein is one you have. Remain positive and remember while reading this book that you are unique. Just as every stroke, cancer, diabetes and heart disease patient is different, so is every postcholecystectomy patient.

So, what qualifies me to write a book on postcholecystectomy syndrome? First, I have lived with postcholecystectomy syndrome for nearly two decades. I have scoured the Internet for a diagnosis and cure. I have read countless research articles about postcholecystectomy syndrome, most of which I cite throughout this book.

Second, I have been a member and administrator of postcholecystectomy support groups for many years. I have found the most valuable information about my symptoms and conditions did not come from my doctors. Instead, much of the information in this book came from other patients. It may not be the most evidence-based way of delivering information, but is proven and helpful.

Since there are numerous conditions linked to cholecystectomy, my goal was to describe all the potential problems that could arise from gallbladder surgery. Patients also needed a roadmap to diagnosis, treatment, diet, finding a doctor and accessing support.

Many of you reading this book have no clue what is causing your symptoms and have doctors who may not believe in postcholecystectomy syndrome. Yes, unfortunately, there are doctors who believe the gallbladder is useless and nothing could possibly go wrong once it is removed. However, since your symptoms occurred following gallbladder surgery, you know there *must* be a link.

Having a mystery condition incited fear and frustration in me for a very long time. Once I linked my symptoms to the fact I had no gallbladder, I could put the pieces together. Therefore, simply picking up this book shows you have gotten past the most important first step—knowing you have postcholecystectomy syndrome.

There isn't a shred of doubt that all my digestive issues over the past 18 years developed as the result of my cholecystectomy. At the very least, the cholecystectomy triggered conditions I may have had all along or, possibly, created new issues I never had prior to the surgery.

Hopefully, by reading this book, you will learn the exact nature of your condition and how to manage your symptoms. Even if you never get an official name to the cause of your symptoms, you can still utilize natural or prescription remedies to provide relief.

Most of you reading this have already had your gallbladder removed. If you still have your gallbladder, I encourage you to seek alternate remedies for dealing with your gallbladder issues, unless your gallbladder is completely full of gallstones, severely diseased or you have gallbladder cancer.

Chapter 1: About the Gallbladder

Contrary to popular belief, our gallbladder is an important organ with very important functions. It is a storage tank, cleanser, and vessel for delivering bile, which is essential for digesting fats and proteins. Prior to having my gallbladder removed, I trusted my surgeon when he told me I needed gallbladder surgery. After my surgery, while I was in the hospital's recovery room, the surgeon said he was convinced I made the right choice, that my gallbladder was full of stones and upon removal looked diseased.

Having done extensive research about cholecystectomy, I now question if I truly needed this organ removed. I suppose I will never know for sure. At the time, I did not think of questioning my doctor. He had an "MD" at the end of his name and went to college for a bunch of years. He was the expert. I was the patient who knew very little about the medical field.

I feel differently today and believe the patient is an "expert," at least regarding their own health and symptomology. After the health experiences I went through, I learned it was important to educate myself on conditions and question everything a doctor tells me, obtaining a second and third opinion when surgeries and procedures are recommended.

You may be wondering, "You mean my doctor does not have my best interest at heart?" No, I am not saying that. What I am saying is that today's medical profession is more apt to perform surgeries and prescribe medications rather than look to alternative health solutions. They often treat the symptoms rather than getting to the exact nature of what is causing the symptoms or seek a holistic route. I don't think doctors intend to do harm. In fact, every doctor swears on the Hippocratic Oath, "to do no harm." They are simply employing what they have learned through years of schooling.

My experience from meeting other postcholecystectomy patients, and doing my own research, is that when a patient has disabling symptoms, and the gallbladder could be the cause, doctors rush to remove it, often with the hope the patient's symptoms will be resolved.

Cholecystectomy, is primarily an elective surgery, meaning the patient elects to have the surgery performed. Patients often don't know they are electing to have this organ removed and that, in some cases, is not a life or death surgery. Most cholecystectomy patients would not die if their gallbladders weren't removed. However, when symptoms disrupt daily life, patients may opt for a cholecystectomy.

With the advent of laparoscopic surgery in the late 80s/early 90s, gallbladders are removed more than ever before. This is likely due to the minimally invasive outpatient nature of these surgeries. Prior to the advent of laparoscopic surgery, the only way a surgeon could remove a gallbladder was through open abdominal surgery, known as a laparotomy, which is a surgical procedure involving a large incision through the abdominal wall to gain access into the abdominal cavity.

Laparotomy requires a very long recovery period as several layers of skin and muscle are cut. Laparoscopic surgery is a technique in which a surgery is conducted using small incisions and a laparoscope. The laparoscope has a camera so the surgeon can see clearly the area he must operate since it is beneath the skin, muscle, and possibly other organs. Many complex laparoscopic surgeries today use a robot to make incisions and access areas a surgeon's hands cannot.

There are many advantages to laparoscopic surgery versus laparotomy. Pain. Bleeding, and scarring are reduced due to smaller incisions and recovery times are often shorter. Laparotomy has the potential for greater complications, a large scar, higher chance for abdominal adhesions (scar tissue), long inpatient hospital stays, and a much greater recovery period.

The following image depicts the difference between a laparoscopic cholecystectomy and an open cholecystectomy (laparotomy).

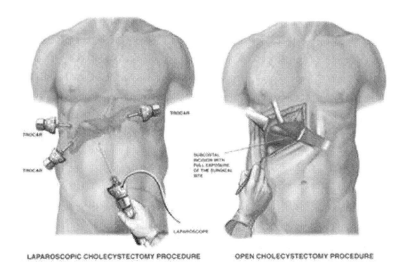

LAPAROSCOPIC CHOLECYSTECTOMY PROCEDURE   OPEN CHOLECYSTECTOMY PROCEDURE

Though 600,000 patients are treated with cholecystectomies every year in the U.S, the American College of Physicians formally advises a conservative "wait and see" approach to gallbladder diseases as cholecystecomy surgery is not without risks.

A study following 9,542 cholecystectomy patients over nine years found these risks: hemorrhage (224 cases, 2.3%), iatrogenic perforation of the gallbladder (1517 cases, 15.9%) and common bile duct (CBD) injuries (17 cases, 0.1%). Conversion to open abdominal operation was necessary in 184 patients (1.9%), due to patient anatomy and/or significant inflammation of the gallbladder. The main postoperative complications were bile leakage (54 cases), hemorrhage (15 cases), sub-hepatic abscess (10 cases) and retained bile duct stones (11 cases). Ten deaths were recorded (0.1%).

In my opinion, removing 600,000 gallbladders a year is beyond excessive. There aren't enough long-term studies showing how the removal of this organ not only affects bile production and release, but also its long-term effect on the liver, surrounding organs, sphincter of Oddi, nervous system, and our body's innate manner of digesting foods.

For example, if you are 35-years-old at the time of cholecystectomy, your body has learned over a 35-year period a certain way of digesting foods in its own symbiotic manner. An interruption or change in your natural digestive process will take some adjusting.

Though I know many people with no postcholecystectomy symptoms or problems, I know many more struggling with symptoms ranging from mild to severe. These people have told me they wished they never had their gallbladders removed. Some don't even know why they had their gallbladders removed.

I conducted a poll through The Sphincter of Oddi Dysfunction Awareness and Education Network, where, astonishingly, 9.5% of respondents didn't know why their gallbladders had been removed. Nearly 60% had conditions that likely qualified for non-surgical gallbladder treatments.

Applying these statistics to that large 600,000 number, assuming these individuals could avert cholecystectomy, only 183,000 cholecystectomies would be necessary each year. Imagine the insurance and copays saved, complications avoided, and work hours retained.

Not only might there be non-surgical solutions to a patient's gallbladder issues, patients may have never had anything wrong with their gallbladder in the first place. This happened to a friend of mine. She went through a rough time with debilitating digestive symptoms. Bloodwork and scans were fairly normal, though her second home became the emergency room. She had a HIDA scan which showed her gallbladder was functioning well. Scans showed no sign of gallstones or gallbladder disease. Regardless, a surgeon convinced her to have her gallbladder removed on the chance it might make her feel better and resolve her mysterious symptoms.

I was shocked and encouraged her to not have it removed. My friend went through with the surgery, but continued to have the same symptoms with the added bonus of bile diarrhea due to the cholecystectomy. Eventually, her symptoms improved. I believe this was because she healed from whatever afflicted her in the first place, which probably was not the gallbladder. That is just my opinion and not a medical fact.

Questions I would love answered are, "How do these doctors and hospitals get the health insurance companies to approve removing an organ when there is zero sign of it needing to be removed when less invasive treatments could be trialed?" Furthermore, "How do these doctors and hospitals justify removing someone's organ, providing little to no information about postcholecystectomy complications?" I am yet to meet a single person with postcholecystectomy issues who was informed by their doctors about all the possible complications of gallbladder surgery.

I am not advocating for anyone to not listen to their doctor. Just be informed. I would not have an organ removed ever again unless I knew it had to be removed—that my life depended on it. Yes, some gallbladders are so diseased and full of stones they must be removed. Some people have gallbladder cancer. And, yes, most cholecystectomy patients do feel better afterward.

If you are reading this and have not had a cholecystectomy, rather than roll the dice, ask your doctor about these potential treatments to circumvent surgery:

Endoscopic Retrograde Cholangiopancreatography (ERCP): a non-surgical procedure used to remove stones, sludge, treat SOD, place stents or apply balloon dilatation to widen the bile duct, and use special x-rays for diagnostic purposes.

Extracorporeal Shock Wave Lithotripsy (ESWL): uses high-frequency sound waves to shatter cholesterol gallstones into pieces small enough to pass through the bile ducts into the intestines.

Ursodiol: a medication that suppresses cholesterol production in the liver, reducing the amount of cholesterol in bile, which can cause gallstones.

Natural Treatments: seek out a natural health practitioner to get your hormones in check naturally and prescribe supplements, herbs, dietary changes, and other natural treatments.

What is the Gallbladder and What Does It Do?

The gallbladder is a pear-shaped organ the size of a small potato that sits beneath the liver just under the right ribcage. It is attached to the liver's biliary system to the cystic duct and stores bile, a liquid produced by the liver, in its hollow sac-like chamber. The gallbladder stores concentrated bile until it is needed to digest foods.

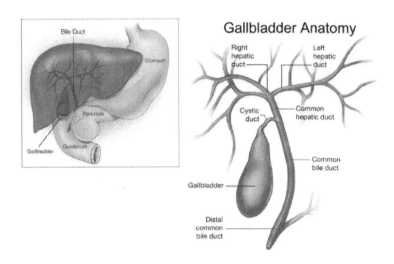

Bile is typically a greenish-to-brownish colored fluid. The liver produces about a quart of bile a day. It is composed of water, cholesterol, phospholipids (type of fat), bile salts, proteins and bilirubin (the product of hemoglobin from the blood after it is broken down in the liver). Bile also contains waste products the liver detoxified.

Bile is essential for removing cholesterol, bilirubin, and toxins from our body. It is essentially a detergent for chemicals, medications, and impurities of one kind or another. Even polluted air is ultimately detoxified through the liver and exits via bile. Bile also, through its action on gut and intestinal motility (a term used to describe the contraction of the muscles that mix and propel contents in the gastrointestinal tract), reduces the number of bacteria found in the small intestine and biliary tract to prevent bacterial overgrowth.

Bile is concentrated by the gallbladder, where most of the water content is removed. This is a very important function as too much water in the bile will impede the body's ability to properly digest fats. If bile is overly concentrated, gallstones may form.

For digestive purposes, the most important component of bile is bile salts, which are acidic compounds that break down fats or make them water-soluble, as oily substances repel water. Bile salts make up about 80% of bile. They are made up of cholesterol (cholic and chenodeoxycolic acids) that have amino acids added to them (glycine or taurine) to form taurocholic acid and glycocholic acid. They are called "salts" because there is an extra positive sodium ion attached to each molecule.

Bile is essential to digesting fats and proteins, as protein- and fatty-rich foods are more difficult to digest than carbohydrates. Imagine trying to wash a greasy pan with just water and no dish soap. In this sense, bile is a sort of detergent, cleaning up and breaking down fats. The transformation of fats by bile salts in the duodenum is also important for preparing and emulsifying fat-soluble vitamins (A, E, D, and K) to pass through the lining of the intestine into the bloodstream.

When food is digested in the stomach, it mixes with stomach acid and becomes "chyme" (another word for partially digested food). Chyme from the stomach enters the duodenum (first part of the small intestine) and contains receptors that monitor the chemical makeup of chyme. When these receptors detect proteins or fats, they produce a hormone called cholecystokinin (CCK).

CCK enters the bloodstream and travels to the gallbladder where it stimulates the smooth muscle tissue in the walls of the gallbladder. CCK triggers the muscles of the gallbladder to contract. The greater amount of fat or protein in a meal, the more CCK will react. This forces the gallbladder to empty bile into the cystic duct and then to the common bile duct. Bile meets up with chyme after passing through the sphincter of Oddi and into the duodenum. See figure below.

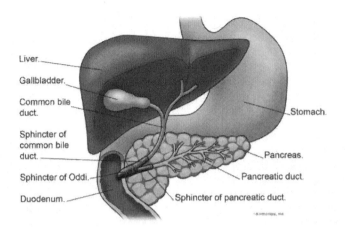

When not receiving a stimulus from the CCK in the duodenum, which is pretty much the same as the time between meals (with a lag for digestion), the bile diverts to the gallbladder for storage to be used later when a meal is ingested.

Large amounts of bile acids are secreted into the intestine every day, but only relatively small quantities are lost from the body. This is because approximately 95% of the bile acids delivered to the duodenum are absorbed back into the blood within the ileum (the last part of the small intestine). There it is transported back to the liver. The net effect of this recirculation is that each bile salt molecule is reused about 20 times, often two or three times during a single digestive phase.

For the sake of review, bile (www.liverdoctor.com):

--Enables fat digestion
--Enables absorption of fat-soluble antioxidants and vitamins A, E, D and K
--Assists the removal of cholesterol from your body
--Assists the removal of toxins that have been broken down by the liver

Things that Can Go Wrong with Your Gallbladder

Just like any other organ in the human body, your gallbladder can develop problems. Though not every gallbladder disease warrants removal of the organ, treatment of the symptoms and underlying condition must be addressed.

Gallstones

Gallstones can occur in the gallbladder, bile duct, and even the entrance to the pancreatic duct. They are not actually stones but can be hard like a stone. The formation of gallstones is often preceded by the presence of biliary sludge, a viscous mixture of glycoproteins, calcium deposits, and cholesterol crystals in the gallbladder or biliary ducts. Gallstones can be as small as a grain of sand and as large as a golf ball.

About 20 million people in the USA (15% of the population) have gallstones. People can have gallstones and not know it, experiencing no symptoms. However, if a gallstone blocks the biliary or pancreatic duct, signs and symptoms may include:

Pain in the upper right portion of your abdomen or below the sternum in the center of the abdomen.
Back pain between your shoulder blades or radiating up your right shoulder.
Yellowing of the skin and the white part of the eyes (jaundice).
Dark urine.
Light-colored, white or clay-colored stools.
A fever and chills.

There are two primary forms of gallstones—cholesterol and pigment stones. Cholesterol stones are usually yellow-green in color. According to Johns Hopkins Medicine, they are the most common type, accounting for 80% of gallstones. Cholesterol gallstones typically develop when bile contains too much cholesterol and not enough bile salts.

Two other factors may cause cholesterol gallstones. The first is the inability of the gallbladder to contract and empty in a timely manner. The second is the presence of proteins in the liver and bile that either promote or inhibit cholesterol crystallization into gallstones. In addition, increased levels of the hormone estrogen, because of pregnancy or hormone therapy, or the use of combined (estrogen-containing) forms of hormonal contraception, may increase cholesterol levels in bile and decrease gallbladder movement, resulting in gallstone formation.

Pigment stones are smaller and darker and usually numerous. They are composed primarily of excess bilirubin and calcium salts that are found in bile. They do contain a small amount of cholesterol. Reasons why your liver makes too much bilirubin include liver cirrhosis, biliary tract infections, and certain blood disorders.

According to the Mayo Clinic, factors that may increase your risk of gallstones include:

Being female
Being age 60 or older
Being an American Indian
Being a Mexican-American
Being overweight or obese
Being pregnant
Eating a high-fat diet
Eating a high-cholesterol diet
Eating a low-fiber diet
Having a family history of gallstones
Having diabetes
Losing weight very quickly
Taking some cholesterol-lowering medications
Taking medications that contain estrogen, such as hormone therapy drugs.

Estrogen is the reason women are more likely to develop gallstones than men as estrogen has been known to increase cholesterol levels in bile and decrease gallbladder function. Pregnancy and hormone replacement therapy, including birth control, increases a woman's risk due to rising estrogen levels.

If you are overweight or obese, your cholesterol levels may be elevated and make it harder for the gallbladder to empty completely. Conversely, if you lose weight or fast, your liver will make extra cholesterol, and your gallbladder may not contract as much.

Diabetes can increase the risk of gallstones as people with this condition often have higher levels of triglycerides (a type of blood fat). If you take medicine to lower your cholesterol, it will increase the amount of cholesterol in bile, which could increase your chances of getting cholesterol stones.

Another reason gallstones occur is when your gallbladder doesn't empty completely or often enough. This causes bile to become very concentrated, contributing to the formation of gallstones. Therefore, if your gallbladder is functioning in an optimal manner, you may have these risk factors, yet gallstones will not form.

Cholecystitis (Inflammation of the Gallbladder)

Cholecystitis is the most common type of gallbladder disease. It presents itself as either an acute or chronic inflammation of the gallbladder. In most cases, gallstones blocking the duct leading out of your gallbladder cause cholecystitis. This results in bile buildup that can cause inflammation. Other potential causes of cholecystitis include bile duct problems, infection, and tumors.

Acute cholecystitis is generally caused by gallstones, but it may also be the result of tumors or various other illnesses. It may present with pain in the upper right side or upper middle part of the abdomen. The pain tends to occur right after a meal and ranges from a sharp stabbing pain to a dull ache that can radiate to your right shoulder. Acute cholecystitis can also cause fever, nausea, vomiting, jaundice, and different colored stools.

Chronic cholecystitis can occur after several attacks of acute cholecystitis. These repeated acute attacks cause the gallbladder to atrophy and lose its ability to effectively store and release bile. Abdominal pain, nausea, and vomiting may occur.

Functional Gallbladder Disorder

The nature of functional gallbladder disorder is unclear, but it is generally regarded as a motility disorder of the gallbladder. In other words, the gallbladder does not contract or function properly. It may result from an initial metabolic disorder, which is any condition that results in problems with metabolism, the process your body uses to get or make energy from the food you eat.

Functional gallbladder disorder may also stem from bile supersaturated with cholesterol or a primary motility disorder in the absence, at least initially, of any abnormalities of bile composition. It has been noted that patients with functional gallbladder disorder may have abnormal stomach emptying and colonic transit, where the stomach and/or small and large intestines empty too quickly or too slowly.

The motility disorder of the gallbladder is called gallbladder dyskinesia. Motility disorder of the sphincter of Oddi is called sphincter of Oddi dysfunction (SOD). This disorder is categorized as two distinct types—biliary sphincter of Oddi dysfunction and pancreatic sphincter of Oddi dysfunction. Patients with either of these conditions present with biliary-type pain, and investigations show no evidence of gallstones in the gallbladder. Biliary dyskinesia is a functional/motility disorder that affects the gallbladder and sphincter of Oddi.

Functional gallbladder disorder is a diagnosis of exclusion in a patient with typical biliary-type pain. The first step in the evaluation of such patients is to exclude other causes for the patient's pain. If no other causes are identified, patients should undergo a cholecystokinin (CCK)-stimulated cholescintigraphy (also known as a nuclear HIDA scan) to confirm the diagnosis. CCK-stimulated cholescintigraphy allows for calculation of the gallbladder ejection fraction (GBEF), which is low in patients with functional gallbladder disorder and helps predict which patients are likely to respond to cholecystectomy.

Pancreatitis

Cholecystectomy is sometimes performed when a patient has recurrent episodes of acute pancreatitis, where the pancreas suddenly becomes inflamed. Surgical removal of the gallbladder is often recommended during the same admission in mild cases to prevent a recurrence. In patients with severe biliary pancreatitis (usually caused by gallstones), it is generally accepted to perform an interventional cholecystectomy. Some patients never have issues with their pancreas again once the gallbladder is removed while others develop chronic pancreatitis, which is chronic inflammation of the pancreas.

Gallbladder Cancer

Gallbladder cancer is usually not found at an early stage because the gallbladder is located deep inside the body and sometimes there may be no symptoms at all. Therefore, gallbladder cancer can be difficult to detect during routine physical examinations.

Sometimes, gallbladder cancer is found unexpectedly after removal of the gallbladder for another reason, such as gallstones. Gallbladder cancer is generally uncommon.

Other Reasons for Gallbladder Removal

As I mentioned earlier, some doctors remove gallbladders without any evidence of gallstones, disease, or a functional disorder. It is a surgery of exclusion to see if cholecystectomy will resolve mystery symptoms. In some cases, the surgery helps. In others, it does nothing, worsens symptoms, or causes new symptoms to arise.

Chapter 2: Postcholecystectomy Syndrome

Obviously, you can survive without a gallbladder. Otherwise, cholecystectomy would not be such a common surgery. However, surviving without an organ and living a healthy life without it are two very different things. After a cholecystectomy, you are more prone to develop certain health problems. For example, you are at greater risk of developing a fatty liver, diarrhea, constipation, biliary issues, indigestion and developing deficiencies of essential fatty acids and fat-soluble nutrients.

Gallbladder functions described in the previous chapter are no longer in play. Bile is no longer stored and concentrated, which can lead to unpleasant symptoms. When your body is void of a gallbladder, bile freely flows from the liver to the bile duct, exiting through the sphincter of Oddi into the duodenum. The high-water content of bile is no longer removed, and overly concentrated bile is not conjugated in the gallbladder.

Change in bile chemistry isn't the only thing that occurs after cholecystectomy. Surgeries are never perfect or fool-proof. Therefore, human error can bring about injury to the ducts. Adhesions (scar tissue) can form following surgery, and some people are more prone to developing them. Also, dramatic changes may occur within the liver itself due to the absence of a gallbladder.

The following is a graphic of anatomy before cholecystectomy and after.

Cholecystectomy

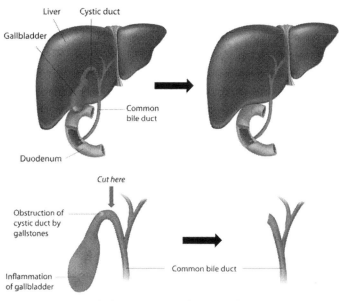

Cholecystectomy Before and After

Any health issues or symptoms arising because of gallbladder removal is called postcholecystectomy syndrome. Postcholecystectomy syndrome describes the appearance of symptoms after cholecystectomy. It is widely estimated 10-15% of the population experience some form of postcholecystectomy syndrome, but Merck Manual estimates anywhere from 5-40% of cholecystectomy patients experience some form of symptoms following cholecystectomy.

Considering these estimates, it is ironic and unsettling that a seemingly disposable organ could wreak such havoc on our bodies once it is removed. This vague yet broad range of suspected postcholecystectomy syndrome patients indicates the need for more research regarding this syndrome.

The most common causes of postcholecystectomy syndrome relate to the change in bile flow and concentration, complications from surgery (i.e. adhesions, cystic duct remnant, common duct injury), retained gallstones or microscopic gallstones, effect on sphincter of

Oddi function, and excessive bile that is malabsorbed in the intestines.

Possible Conditions Linked to Postcholecystectomy Syndrome

Jensen, et al described in their research paper, *Postcholecystectomy Syndrome,* over 60 different potential causes of and links to postcholecystectomy syndrome, broken down by anatomy. The following is a list of those etiologies with definitions. Some overlap and are repetitive in nature. Some you may question how postcholecystectomy syndrome could possibly be linked to the associated condition, i.e. brain and nervous system health. Keep in mind your digestive system is integral to keeping your entire body running smoothly and feeling great.

Some of these conditions are rare or inconclusive relative to postcholecystectomy syndrome. Therefore, please do not read the following conditions and think you have or will develop the more life-threatening conditions listed. Also, as I recommended previously, don't self-diagnose. Instead, share this information with your health care provider.

Gallbladder remnant and cystic duct

Residual or reformed gallbladder—usually occurs when a full cholecystectomy is not performed, due to various reasons, and part of the gallbladder remains. Even the smallest gallbladder remnant can cause cystic duct lesions and biliary sludge. Common symptoms are right upper quadrant pain and nausea or vomiting. If symptoms are severe or there is a blockage, a repeat cholecystectomy is needed to remove the remnant gallbladder and/or shorten the cystic duct.

Stump cholelithiasis—gallstones or calculi (very small gallstone particles) lodged in the remaining cystic duct. Common symptoms are right upper quadrant pain and nausea or vomiting. If there is a blockage, treatments may include laparoscopic surgery or endoscopic retrograde cholangiopancreatography (ERCP) to remove the debris. Ursodeoxycholic acid may be prescribed to thin the bile.

Neuroma—pinched nerve or benign nerve tumor that usually involves the intercostal nerve (nerves from the spine to the ribs). This can occur as a trauma from surgery. Patients generally experience pain to the touch of their right rib area and may feel a burning sensation that often spreads to the back and shoulder. Treatment typically involves nerve pain medication, nerve block injections, and/or surgical resection of the intercostal nerve.

Liver

Fatty infiltration of liver—also known as fatty liver, non-alcoholic fatty liver disease (NAFD), or steatohepatitis. Following gallbladder removal, individuals may not conjugate adequate bile salts, which are needed to properly digest and store fats. Subsequently, some of the fat a cholecystectomy patient ingests ends up in the liver. Although it is normal for the liver to contain a small amount of fat, too much fat in the liver may contribute to insulin sensitivity and liver inflammation, which could inhibit bile production and progress to scarring and irreversible damage. Most patients with fatty liver are asymptomatic (no symptoms), but some experience enlarged liver, upper right quadrant pain, and fatigue. The main course of treatment focuses on dietary changes, weight loss, and exercise.

Hepatitis—a liver infection brought on by extrahepatic (outside liver) and intrahepatic (inside liver) bile duct dilatation (widening/enlargement of the bile duct) following cholecystectomy. It may also be related to bile duct injury during cholecystectomy. Hepatitis symptoms include jaundice (yellowing of eyes and skin), fatigue, fever, diarrhea, abdominal pain, nausea, and headaches. Treatments involve bed rest and anti-viral medications.

Hydrohepatosis— This is an outdated term referring to dilatation of the intrahepatic bile ducts. This condition is rare and most often involves biliary sludge or a gallstone lodged in an intrahepatic duct. Patients may experience compensatory dilatation of the common bile duct after cholecystectomy because the gallbladder bile pool disappears and the buffer storage function is lost. (Source: Lv, Y.) Symptoms include pain in the right side, fever, and/or weight loss. Treatment may rely on a wait and see approach. Alternatively, an ERCP or surgery may be required to clean out the duct or place a T-tube for better drainage.

Cirrhosis—a chronic progressive disease of the liver tissue and cells. In cholecystectomy patients, cirrhosis is unlikely but may occur after chronic infections, biliary obstructions, fatty liver progression, or scar tissue build up. Symptoms include fatigue, bleeding and/or bruising easily, itchy skin, jaundice, nausea, loss of appetite, and/or fluid accumulation in the abdomen and elsewhere in the body. Treatment focuses on correcting the underlying cause of the cirrhosis. In severe cases, liver transplant is necessary.

Chronic idiopathic jaundice— a condition in which a person's skin and the whites of the eyes are discolored yellow due to an increased level of bile pigments, specifically conjugated bilirubin, in the blood. Idiopathic means jaundice occurs for unknown reasons. However, for cholecystectomy patients, jaundice may occur due to changes in bile conjugation. In addition to yellowing, jaundice may cause fatigue, nausea, pruritus (itchy skin), pale stools, weight loss, and/or vomiting. Treatment is conservative, involving dietary changes and medications.

Gilbert disease (Gilbert syndrome)—generally, a harmless liver condition in which the liver doesn't properly process bilirubin. It is caused by a genetic variant and not cholecystectomy. However, Gilbert disease may be exacerbated by cholecystectomy in patients who have this genetic variant. The primary symptom is yellowing of the skin and eyes. There is no recommended treatment for this disease.

Dubin-Johnson syndrome—a rare, autosomal recessive (inherited from DNA), benign disorder that causes an isolated increase of conjugated bilirubin in the serum. Like Gilbert disease, this disorder is inherited, but symptoms may pronounce after cholecystectomy. Jaundice and abdominal pain are most common symptoms. There is no recommended treatment for this disease.

Hepatolithiasis—the presence of gallstones in the biliary ducts of the liver. Gallstones can form in the intrahepatic ducts of the liver. They may also form outside of the liver but travel back up to an intrahepatic duct. Many with this condition are asymptomatic, but those who have symptoms experience pain in right side, fevers, and/or jaundice. Surgical treatment may be necessary.

Sclerosing cholangitis—a disease of the bile ducts that causes inflammation and fibrosis (scarring and destruction) of bile ducts inside and/or outside of the liver. This is a progressive disease with no known cure. It can impede the flow of bile to the intestines and lead to cirrhosis of the liver, liver failure, and other complications, including bile duct and liver cancer. There are numerous symptoms, including pruritus (itching), fatigue, jaundice, and dark urine. Treatments include ursodeoxycholic acid, cholestyramine, ERCP balloon dilatation, and in severe cases liver transplant.

Cyst—a closed capsule or sac-like structure, typically filled with liquid, semisolid or gaseous material, very much like a blister. Cystic lesions of the liver include the following: simple cysts, multiple cysts arising in the setting of polycystic liver disease (PCLD), parasitic or hydatid (echinococcal) cysts, cystic tumors, and abscesses. Most are asymptomatic and benign. Those that become very large or malignant need to be removed via surgery.

Internal Anatomy of Liver

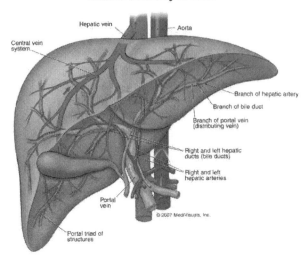

Biliary Tract

Cholangitis—bacterial build up in the bile duct leading to inflammation and infection. After cholecystectomy, bile may not freely flow to counteract bacterial flora making its way up the bile duct from the small intestine. Symptoms include fever, nausea, pruritus, and pain. Standard treatment is an antibiotic. ERCP may also be necessary to clean out the bile duct.

Adhesions—buildup of scar tissue. Adhesions following gallbladder removal are primarily in the cystic duct where the gallbladder was surgically removed. These adhesions can travel and block the common bile duct. Symptoms include upper right quadrant pain, nausea, vomiting, and light-colored stools. If the scar tissue impedes the flow of bile, surgery is needed to remove the adhesions.

Strictures—narrowing of the biliary ducts. Strictures may occur due to adhesions, surgical duct injury, or for unknown reasons. Symptoms depend on the cause of the stricture, but many patients are asymptomatic. Treatments include addressing the root cause of the stricture or an ERCP with balloon dilatation.

Trauma—this refers to any injury to the bile duct because of cholecystectomy surgery. Mistakes can occur during surgery, including accidentally nicking the bile duct. If this happens, a bile leak will occur, and symptoms range from pain to nausea and vomiting. Surgical treatment is required to repair surgical errors.

Cyst—as described earlier, cysts can form in the biliary system as well as the liver. They are generally uncommon and benign. However, if they are large, can become obstructive and need to be removed.

Malignancy and cholangiocarcinoma—another term for bile duct cancer. Bile duct cancer is composed of mutated epithelial (tissue) cells (or cells showing characteristics of epithelial differentiation) and can occur in the intrahepatic or extrahepatic biliary tissue. There are typically no symptoms until the disease has progressed, at which point symptoms may include pruritus, jaundice, pain, loss of appetite and weight loss, nausea/vomiting, dark urine, light colored stool, and fever. Treatment depends on whether the cancer can be removed through surgery. If not, then treatments for cancer like radiation and chemotherapy are recommended.

Obstruction—the bile duct can become obstructed with gallstones or biliary microlesia (sludge), food particles, or adhesions. Symptoms are jaundice, nausea/vomiting, upper right quadrant pain, fever, constipation/diarrhea, and/or light-colored stools. Treatment depends on the cause of the obstruction, but usually requires medications like ursodeoxycholic acid, an ERCP, or surgery.

Choledocholithiasis—the presence of at least one gallstone in the biliary duct. Symptoms and treatment are the same for an obstruction.

Dilation without obstruction—this is often related to problems with the sphincter of Oddi or from biliary sludge. Symptoms and treatment coincide with sphincter of Oddi dysfunction (discussed later). For biliary sludge, symptoms are similar for obstruction and are treated with medications, dietary changes, and/or ERCP.

Hypertension or nonspecific dilation—abnormally high blood pressure in the portal vein (the large vein that brings blood from the intestine to the liver) and its branches. Alternatively, this refers to any elevated pressure of the bile duct. Most patients are asymptomatic, but biliary hypertension has been linked to bouts of pancreatitis. Most common symptom is upper right quadrant pain. There is no recommended treatment.

Dyskinesia—recurrent right upper quadrant pain in the absence of gallstones often caused by a motility disorder of the biliary system. In general, biliary dyskinesia is the disturbance in the coordination of contraction of the biliary ducts, and/or reduction in the speed of emptying of the biliary tree into the duodenum. In addition to pain, symptoms may include nausea/vomiting, weight loss, and constipation/diarrhea. Treatments include anti-spasmodic medications, ERCP, and in severe cases biliary roux en y surgery to re-route the bile duct.

Fistula—A biliary fistula is a type of fistula (an abnormal connection between two hollow places) in which bile flows along an abnormal connection from the bile ducts into a nearby hollow structure. The likelihood of a fistula forming is rare and is usually attributed to a postcholecystectomy surgical error. The only treatment is to surgically correct the fistula. Symptoms are the same for an obstruction.

Periampullary—any issue, including carcinoma (tissue cancer), of the ampulla of Vater (entrance from the duodenum to the bile and pancreatic ducts). Polyps, cysts, and tumors can present in this area. Symptoms are generally benign. However, if the growth causes an obstruction, bile and pancreatic fluids cannot flow out to the small intestine. Symptoms are the same as an obstruction, but could also cause pancreatitis. An ERCP or surgery is required if there is an obstruction. If the growth is cancerous and cannot be surgically removed, radiation and chemotherapy treatment may be necessary.

Sphincter of Oddi dysfunction (SOD), spasm, or hypertrophy—this is a controversial and complicated condition. It is difficult to diagnose as most patients have normal bloodwork and scan results.

For unknown reasons, SOD is most common in women who had their gallbladders removed. Symptoms are upper right quadrant pain (often severe), nausea/vomiting, weight loss, and/or diarrhea/constipation. Treatments include medications, ERCP with sphincterotomy (cutting the sphincter of Oddi and/or biliary and pancreatic sphincters), and surgery.

Sphincter of Oddi stricture—narrowing of the sphincter of Oddi. Symptoms and treatments are similar to periampullary issues and SOD.

Papilloma—a small wart-like growth that can appear at the end of the bile duct. Symptoms and treatments similar to periampullary issues.

Cancer—any form of bile duct cancer due to changes in biliary environment. See "malignancies" above.

Pancreas

Pancreatitis—any inflammation of the pancreas. There are two types: acute and chronic. Gallstones, biliary sludge, and/or pancreatic stones (small "stones" that develop from calcium deposits in the pancreas) all can block the flow of digestive enzymes from the pancreas to the small intestine. This will cause inflammation in the pancreas. Symptoms are abdominal pain (often unbearable), nausea/vomiting, fever, weight loss, and diarrhea/constipation or greasy stools. Treatment may require hospitalization for fluids and antibiotics. Food and drink is withheld during acute episodes. For chronic pancreatitis, treatment includes pain control, digestive enzymes, stents, and surgery or removal of the pancreas.

Pancreatic cancer—a malignant cancer that forms in the tissues of the pancreas and has a poor prognosis. Symptoms are similar to pancreatitis but may also include biliary symptoms if a tumor affects the bile duct. Treatment is typical of any cancer treatment—chemotherapy, radiation, and/or surgery.

Pancreatic cysts—there are generally two main varieties of pancreatic cysts based on the type of fluid they contain. The most common cysts are either serous (containing a thin type of fluid) or mucinous (containing a thicker, more viscous fluid). These cysts can be benign, but can cause inflammation and become infected. They may also impede the release of pancreatic enzymes. Treatment includes antibiotics, pain control, digestive enzymes, withholding food and drink, and/or surgery.

Benign tumors—a non-malignant growth of endocrine or exocrine cells in the pancreas. Symptoms are similar to pancreatic cancer. Treatment may include doing nothing or performing surgery to remove the tumor.

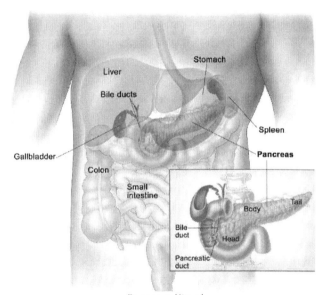

Pancreas Visual

Esophagus

Aerophagia—a condition of excessive air swallowing, which goes to the stomach. This can occur as the result of a changing acid environment in the stomach and esophagus. It is considered a functional disorder. Symptoms include excessive belching, stomach upset and pain, and excessive bloat and flatulence. Treatment should focus on the underlying cause. Symptom management may include antacids and holistic ways to mop up excess air and gas.

Diaphragmatic hernia—a defect or hole in the diaphragm that allows the abdominal contents to move into the chest cavity. This is a rare condition to occur in adulthood. During adult-onset, this condition is almost always caused by trauma, as could happen during cholecystectomy surgery. Symptoms are pain, nausea/vomiting, caved in or protruding stomach, and labored breathing. Treatment is surgery.

Hiatal hernia—occurs when part of your stomach pushes upward through your diaphragm. Most hiatal hernias are asymptomatic, but patients may experience heartburn, belching, difficulty swallowing, chest or abdominal pain, fullness after meals, and nausea/vomiting. Treatment includes antacids and surgery.

Achalasia—disease of the muscle of the lower esophageal body and the lower esophageal sphincter that prevents relaxation of the sphincter and an absence of contractions, or peristalsis, of the esophagus. Symptoms include dysphagia (difficulty in swallowing), regurgitation of undigested food, chest pain behind the sternum, and weight loss. Treatments are lifestyle changes, antacids, esophageal dilatation, and surgery.

Stomach

Bile gastritis—also known as "bile reflux" and occurs when bile backs up (refluxes) into your stomach and esophagus. This can cause a broad range of symptoms like nausea/vomiting, burning pain, reflux, and complications associated with not having enough stomach acid (bile essentially neutralizes stomach acid). A condition called Barrett's esophagus can occur after the esophagus is exposed to bile for prolonged periods. Treatments include sleeping upright or at an angle, cholestyramine, Carafate, gut motility medications, and antacids (although antacids technically do not work on bile reflux). If the cause of bile gastritis is from an anatomical defect, surgery may be needed.

Peptic ulcer disease—refers to a painful open sore or ulcer in the lining of the stomach or duodenum. An H Pylori infection can cause ulcers, as can bile reflux and excessive stomach acid due to inflammation of the stomach lining. Symptoms include nausea, vomiting (sometimes bloody), burning pain, and general stomach upset. Treatments vary depending on the cause of the ulcer. Antibiotics, antacids, Carafate, Pepto Bismol, or PPIs may be prescribed. Lifestyle and dietary changes can help. Surgery is rarely needed.

Gastric cancer—stomach cancer. It is unclear what exactly causes stomach cancer, but it has been linked to inflammation in the gut, smoking, diet and H Pylori infection. Symptoms are stomach pain, nausea/vomiting, weight loss, blood in stool, constipation/diarrhea, weakness, heartburn, trouble swallowing, and stomach swelling. Treatment involves surgery, chemotherapy, and/or radiation.

Duodenum (First Part of Small Intestine)

Adhesions—scar tissue from the cholecystectomy site can spread to the outside of the duodenum. If you ever had an ERCP with sphincterotomy, adhesions can appear where the cut to the sphincter of Oddi was made. Adhesions can be asymptomatic or cause issues similar to an obstruction. Treatment is rarely needed. However, in some instances, surgery is necessary to remove the adhesions.

Duodenal diverticula—pouch-like herniations in the duodenal wall or Papilla of Vater. Symptoms are usually not present but are detected through endoscopy. When symptoms are present, patients may experience upper abdominal pain and pressure, right upper quadrant pain, nausea, vomiting, and if the diverticula obstruct the bile duct, jaundice may be present. Treatment focuses on dietary changes, adding a fiber supplement, and antibiotics. Surgery is reserved for complicated cases.

Irritable bowel disease—more commonly known as irritable bowel syndrome or IBS. IBS is a blanket term for disturbances in bowel function and motility, most of which are idiopathic. IBS of the duodenum is a rare diagnosis. It could refer to any unexplained irritation of the duodenum or disruption in duodenal functions. Symptoms vary depending on the type of irritation or problem. Treatment is generally reserved to medications to relieve symptoms.

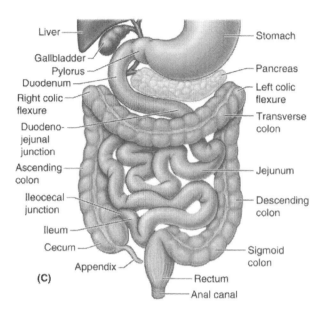

Small Bowel (Jejunum and Ileum)

Adhesions—adhesions can spread from the cholecystectomy site to the small intestines, causing an obstruction and damage to the small intestines. Symptoms may include nausea/vomiting, inability to keep food down, abdominal pain, constipation/diarrhea, and weight loss. For less serious symptoms, dietary and lifestyle changes, antispasmodic medications, fiber, and laxatives may help. In severe cases, surgery may be warranted to remove adhesions.

Incisional hernia—a protrusion of tissue or part of an organ through the bone, muscular tissue, or the membrane by which it is normally contained. This rarely occurs because of cholecystectomy. However, adhesions and injury at a portal site (from laparoscopic surgery) may create a hernia. A bulge may appear in the abdomen, which may come and go. If the hernia creates an obstruction, the same symptoms may occur as with adhesions. Surgery may be needed to repair the hernia. Otherwise, the same treatments for adhesions can be employed.

Irritable bowel disease—also known as Irritable Bowel Syndrome (IBS). IBS of the small bowel is a functional disorder where the contractions of the small intestine are disordered or unsynchronized. This can be caused by an unknown functional issue, a pseudo-obstruction or small intestinal bacteria overgrowth. Symptoms are bloating, pain, nausea, and constipation/diarrhea. Treatment is antibiotics, antispasmodics, IBS-specific medications, fiber, dietary and lifestyle changes, and/or surgical correction of an obstruction.

Colon (Large Intestine)

Constipation—The National Institute of Diabetes and Digestive and Kidney Diseases defines constipation as having fewer than three bowel movements a week; and/or bowel movements with stools that are hard, dry, and small, making them painful or difficult to pass. Chronic constipation is a common postcholecystectomy issue and could be related to a functional disorder or alteration in bile output. Treatment includes laxatives, fiber, dietary changes, exercise, IBS medication, and stool softeners. Surgery may be necessary in rare cases of obstruction.

Diarrhea—an increased frequency in bowel movements that are loose or watery. Excess bile and malabsorption of bile can cause diarrhea as can changes in bowel motility. Treatment includes addressing the underlying cause of diarrhea. If excessive bile is the cause, a bile acid sequestrant like cholestyramine may help. Antispasmodics or anti-diarrheal medications can help abate symptoms. Diet and lifestyle changes are often necessary.

Incisional hernia—as described previously, this rarely occurs because of cholecystectomy. See incisional hernia for small bowel.

Irritable bowel disease—(IBS) of the colon is a functional disorder where the contractions of the large intestine are disordered or unsynchronized. Like IBS of the small intestine, this can be caused by an unknown functional issue, bacteria, or an obstruction.

Symptoms are bloating, cramping, pain, nausea, and constipation/diarrhea. Treatments are antibiotics, antispasmodics, fiber, dietary and lifestyle changes, and surgical correction of an obstruction.

Vascular

Intestinal angina—also known as intestinal ischemia. This occurs when blood flow through the major arteries that supply blood to your intestines slows or stops. One potential cause of this from cholecystectomy is due to an increase in cholesterol deposits. Symptoms include abdominal pain or tenderness, fullness after eating, weight loss, nausea or vomiting, diarrhea, blood in stool, and bloating. Treatment involves stopping medications that constrict your blood vessels, surgery, an angioplasty (a balloon is inflated at the end of a catheter to compress the fatty deposits and stretch the artery), and/or stent placement.

Coronary angina—chest pain or discomfort that occurs if an area of your heart muscle doesn't get enough oxygen-rich blood. Laparoscopy is contraindicated in patients with poor cardiac function. Therefore, coronary angina could occur following cholecystectomy. Treatment includes stents, surgery.

Nerve

Neuroma—previously described in Gallbladder remnant section.

Intercostal neuralgia—previously described in Gallbladder remnant section as neuroma.

Spinal nerve lesions—growths on the spinal nerve, due to trauma or unknown reasons. Research has shown that people with a spinal cord injury have an increased susceptibility to gallstones. The reason for this is unknown. However, I could not find a definitive correlation between spinal nerve lesions and cholecystectomy, though the authors of *Postcholecystectomy Syndrome* list this as a possible condition. Spinal nerve lesion pain usually presents as neuropathy. Lesions can also cause sensory impairment and numbness. Treatments are pain or nerve medication, physical therapy, chiropractic manipulation, and in rare cases, surgery.

Sympathetic imbalance—also known as dysautonomia, which means you have over-reactive nerves in what is called your sympathetic or autonomic nervous system. This part of your nervous system helps regulate all the functions of your body that you don't control consciously, i.e. your digestion, your breathing, your heart rate, your energy metabolism, and your circulation. Symptoms are numerous as your sympathetic nervous system affects so many aspects of your body. Treatments vary but are generally benign, focusing on alleviating symptoms.

Neurosis—a relatively mild mental illness that is not caused by organic disease, involving symptoms of stress (depression, anxiety, obsessive behavior, hypochondria) but not a radical loss of touch with reality. Honestly, I am not sure why cholecystectomy would cause neurosis. However, the gut is "the second brain" due to its content of serotonin, GABA, dopamine, norepinephrine and other chemicals affecting brain health. I suppose issues resulting from cholecystectomy could affect these chemicals and subsequently affect brain health. Psychiatric medication and psychotherapy are the standard treatments.

Psychic tension or anxiety—excessive worry or nervousness ranging from mild to debilitating. It produces symptoms of stress, depression, anxiety, obsessive behavior, and/or hypochondria. See neurosis description.

Bone

Arthritis—painful inflammation of the joints. Arthritis is rarely linked to PCS, but in some situations, could be caused by food sensitivities triggered by PCS, especially gluten intolerance or sensitivity. Arthritis pain can occur in any of the body's joints. Treatments are typically nonsteroidal anti-inflammatory drugs (NSAID), other pain medications, and TNF inhibitors, also known as biologic medications. Dietary and natural remedies can be very beneficial as well.

Other

Adrenal cancer—the adrenals are walnut-sized organs on top of your kidneys that control the production of cortisol, a steroid-based hormone synthesized from cholesterol. Symptoms vary greatly depending on the type of cancer or tumor, and are associated with irregularity of the hormones androgen, estrogen, aldosterone and/or cortisol. Treatment is the same as for other cancers but may also involve therapies to correct hormonal imbalances.

Thyrotoxicosis—an excess of thyroid hormone in the body. Having this condition also means that you have a low level of thyroid stimulating hormone, TSH, in your bloodstream, because the pituitary gland senses that you have "enough" thyroid hormone. If you are thyrotoxic, you may feel nervous or irritable, because all your body's functions are speeding up. Other symptoms include weight loss, excessive urination and/or thirst, heart palpitations, and more. Treatments are anti-thyroid drugs, beta blockers, radioiodine, dietary changes, and surgery.

Organ other than hepatobiliary or pancreatic—cholecystectomy may affect other organs of the body but isn't well-documented.

Foreign bodies, including gallstones and surgical clips—I know a woman who had right side pain for years and was misdiagnosed with SOD. Turned out she had a severe titanium allergy linked to the clips placed on the cystic duct following cholecystectomy. She had the clips removed from her cholecystectomy and has been doing better.

More Conditions Linked to Postcholecystectomy Syndrome

The previous section may seem like an exhaustive list of potential links to postcholecystectomy syndrome. However, I found there were a few conditions missing from this list gathered from my experience interacting with other postcholecystectomy patients.

Small Intestinal Bacteria Overgrowth (SIBO)—when bacteria normally found in the large intestine make its way up to the small intestine, an overgrowth can occur, especially if there is a change in bile production and consistency. Bile helps keep bacteria in check. As we reviewed earlier, bile flow and consistency change after cholecystectomy. Symptoms include abdominal bloating, gas, constipation/diarrhea, abdominal pain, and in advanced cases, there may be vitamin and mineral deficiencies and weight loss. Treatment involves dietary changes, antibiotics, and natural supplements.

Gastroparesis— a condition in which the motility of the muscles in your stomach does not function properly and gastric emptying is delayed. Patients enrolled in a National Institute of Diabetes and the Digestive and Kidney Diseases Gastroparesis Registry showed out of 391 subjects with diabetic or idiopathic gastroparesis, 142 (36%) had a prior cholecystectomy at the time of enrollment. Primary symptoms are nausea, vomiting, full feeling in stomach after a few bites of food, and abdominal pain. Treatments include medications, dietary changes, and, in extreme cases, surgical placement of a neurostimulator implant.

Inflammatory Bowel Disease—not to be confused with IBS, it involves chronic inflammation of all or part of your digestive tract. IBD primarily includes ulcerative colitis and Crohn's disease and is an idiopathic disease caused by a dysregulated immune response to intestinal microflora. Like with SIBO, since bile helps regulate intestinal bacterial flora, cholecystectomy could trigger IBD. Common symptoms are diarrhea, fatigue, fever, abdominal pain, blood in stool, reduced appetite, and weight loss. Treatments are dietary modifications, medications, antibiotics, and in severe cases surgery.

Celiac Disease—a genetically linked autoimmune disorder where eating certain types of grain-based products containing gluten sets off an immune mediated response that causes damage to the small intestine. Approximately 60% of celiac disease sufferers are known to have liver, gallbladder, and/or pancreatic conditions. Conversely, I did not find substantive proof cholecystectomy was a cause of celiac disease or gluten sensitivity. I suppose any significant gut changes, as occurs following cholecystectomy, could trigger a pre-existing celiac condition or gluten sensitivity. Most common symptoms are abdominal pain and bloating. Other symptoms that may arise are vomiting, diarrhea, constipation, fatty stool, weight loss, and behavioral changes. Treatment involves avoiding gluten-containing foods, even trace amounts.

Chapter 3: Obtaining a Diagnosis

You have had your gallbladder removed and either your body has acclimated well or, chances are, you are reading this book because you are experiencing troubling symptoms. Alternatively, you may be reading this book to avoid postcholecystectomy symptoms from appearing. If you aren't experiencing symptoms, you may want to skip this chapter. However, if you are experiencing any symptoms, mild or severe, after cholecystectomy, you likely want to know why you feel the way you do and desire answers.

Diagnosing postcholecystectomy syndrome will depend on your symptoms. As you read in the previous chapter, there are numerous etiologies associated with gallbladder removal. The list of potential symptoms is long. I will focus on diagnostic tests relative to digestive symptoms and common postcholecystectomy conditions. Some of the etiologies listed in the previous chapter are rare and don't necessarily involve the digestive system. I will describe the most common tests your doctor would order for postcholecystectomy syndrome.

Bloodwork

Bloodwork should always be ordered and is generally the first go-to test your doctor will employ. A comprehensive metabolic profile is standard. It will show the status of your liver, kidneys, and electrolytes, ex. potassium, sodium, magnesium, and calcium.

I always recommend asking your doctor to include an order to measure your pancreatic enzyme levels as elevated levels could indicate a problem with the sphincters and ducts. It may also indicate the presence of a gallstone or biliary sludge.

Liver function tests are most common in postcholecystectomy patients since it can show whether there are problems with your liver or bile ducts. The most common measurements are taken for:

Alanine transaminase (ALT)—an enzyme that occurs in large amounts in the liver and helps to process proteins. When your liver is injured or inflamed, the blood level of ALT usually rises.

Aspartate aminotransferase (AST)—an enzyme found inside liver cells. When a blood test detects high levels of this enzyme in your blood, it usually means your liver is injured in some way. However, AST can also be released if heart or skeletal muscle is damaged. For this reason, ALT is usually considered to be more specifically related to liver problems.

Alkaline phosphatase (ALP)—an enzyme that occurs mainly in liver cells next to bile ducts, and in bone. The blood level is raised in some types of liver and bone disease.

Albumin—the main protein made by your liver, which circulates in your bloodstream. The ability to make albumin (and other proteins) is affected in some types of liver disorder. A low level of blood albumin occurs in some liver disorders. It can also occur in people who are malnourished.

Total protein—measures albumin and all other proteins in blood. High levels may indicate inflammation or infection. Low levels are associated with liver disease and malnutrition.

Bilirubin—as mentioned previously, this chemical gives bile its yellow/green color. A high level of "conjugated" bilirubin in your blood will make you appear jaundice and occurs in various liver and bile duct conditions. It is particularly high if the flow of bile is blocked. It can also be raised with hepatitis, liver injury, or long-term alcohol abuse. A high level of "unconjugated" bilirubin occurs when there is excessive breakdown of red blood cells or in those with Gilbert's syndrome.

In addition to these tests, if you have lost weight rapidly, you may want to ask your doctor about having your vitamin and mineral levels checked. Various conditions in the liver, stomach, pancreas, and intestines can cause malabsorption. Therefore, mineral and vitamin deficiencies will not indicate the exact cause or nature of the malabsorption. However, knowing your deficiencies will enable your doctor to treat the deficiency with supplements, intravenous infusions, and/or dietary modifications which could lead to improved symptoms.

Inflammation and autoimmune disease markers may also be measured as autoimmune conditions can cause symptoms of liver disease and intestinal problems. These tests can detect primary biliary cirrhosis, autoimmune liver disease (where the body's immune system attacks the liver), celiac disease, and systemic diseases affecting the gastrointestinal system.

Bloodwork is a starting point and can be disappointing when results are perfectly normal. Too often, doctors interpret normal bloodwork results as meaning there is nothing wrong with the patient. Keep in mind, however, that bloodwork does not always show what is really going on. Some end stage liver cirrhosis patients have perfectly normal liver enzyme levels. More unsettling is most people with pancreatic cancer have perfect bloodwork and scans until tumors develop.

During my worst suffering with postcholecystectomy sphincter of Oddi dysfunction, I weighed 95 pounds (40 pounds under my normal weight) with significant muscle wasting. I was barely able to function due to severe dizziness bordering on fainting much of the time. I was so weak that walking from the car into a doctor's office wore me out. The chronic pain and nausea were debilitating.

Although my blood pressure was very low, my bloodwork was perfectly normal. It made no sense. I learned later on there are literally hundreds, possibly thousands, of diseases that cannot be detected through routine bloodwork and scans. Only very specialized tests can detect some conditions.

Another concern is the interpretation of the results. Too often, doctors may report that a result is normal even though it is just shy of abnormal. I recommend every patient obtain copies of their bloodwork, scans, and procedural results for this very reason.

I was fainting and white as a ghost at one point after my surgery. I saw my ferritin level was dangerously low, an indication I was anemic. My total iron was just shy of being abnormally low. For whatever reason, the nutritional MD overseeing my nutritional status did not take it seriously. I had to advocate persistently for iron infusions. Eventually, I got my iron infusions. Color returned to my face, and I felt much better. On another occasion, my bloodwork showed I was only borderline dehydrated, though I came close to blacking out a few times.

This same doctor didn't think it was a problem because my bloodwork was still within the normal range. I had to go to the emergency room and get fluids and electrolytes several times which helped me feel better and resolved the dizziness. I had to continually advocate for fluids and electrolytes. Remember that bumper sticker, "Question Authority?" Practice that, but in a diplomatic, empowered manner.

Food Allergy and Food Sensitivity Testing

In testing for food allergies or sensitivity, blood is drawn or the skin is pricked and then exposed to a panel of foods and food components. IgE-based testing is considered the gold standard for suspected food allergies. IgE, short for "immunoglobulin E," is the antibody that triggers food allergy symptoms.

The IgE Food Antibody Profile measures levels of antigen-specific IgE to common foods. Positive results will indicate the presence of IgE antibodies to specific foods. This test solely produces results for a true allergy, not a food sensitivity, and negative results do not rule out a food allergy. There is also the potential for a "false positive" test result.

Some conventional and alternative health care practitioners utilize IgG-based testing, which has shown some clinically meaningful results. IgG (Immunoglobulin G), have a longer half-life than the traditional IgE allergy as IgG antibodies can lead to inflammatory processes. IgG-mediated symptoms appear up to three days after the consumption of a trigger food, where IgE-mediated responses are often immediate.

IgG Food Antibody testing is a food sensitivity test which helps identify IgG-mediated food sensitivities. This immunological food sensitivity test measures IgG antibody levels to a variety of foods.

Stool Analysis

Your doctor or natural health practitioner may order a stool analysis, which is a series of tests done on a stool sample to help diagnose certain conditions. It can help screen for colon cancer, diagnose infections caused by bacteria, fungus, or a virus; detect the presence of parasites, check for malabsorption and fat in the stool; and identify diseases of the digestive tract, liver, and pancreas
nausea, vomiting, loss of appetite, bloating, abdominal pain and cramping, and fever.

A stool analysis is collected in a container over the course of a few days and then sent to the laboratory. Laboratory analysis includes microscopic examination, chemical tests, and microbiologic tests. The stool will be checked for color, consistency, amount, shape, odor, and the presence of mucus. The stool may be examined for hidden (occult) blood, fat, meat fibers, bile, white blood cells, and sugars called reducing substances. The pH of the stool also may be measured.

Alternative Tests

One of the best things I did for myself was go to a naturopathic doctor. He ordered a series of alternative tests—most of which were costly and not covered by my insurance. I had a comprehensive stool analysis (broader than a traditional stool analysis), organic acids/metabolic analysis test, and saliva hormone profile. The stool analysis showed, not surprisingly to me, that I had a shortage of pancreatic enzymes.

Also, my "good" gut bacteria levels were low. The organic acids/metabolic analysis test used urine and blood to measure malabsorption and dysbiosis (an imbalance of gut bacteria); cellular energy and mitochondrial metabolism; neurotransmitter metabolism; vitamin deficiencies; and toxin exposure and detoxification need. The results of these tests were consistent with some of my symptoms. The saliva hormone test showed my cortisol was all whacky—too high in the morning and in the evening. My adrenals were in overdrive and fatigued. My progesterone and estrogen were super low as well.

Conventional doctors rarely acknowledge the efficacy of these tests though there is evidence to the contrary in medical journals. Regardless, I recommend exploring these tests particularly to measure nutritional status.

Small Intestinal Bacteria Overgrowth (SIBO) Breath Test

SIBO is not commonly recognized as a cause of postcholecystectomy symptoms. Many doctors aren't even equipped to test for this condition. Where I live, gastroenterologists are prevalent. However, only one local practice tests for SIBO. There are SIBO testing kits you can order online, but I recommend finding a doctor to administer the test.

Some doctors rely on an endoscopy to test for SIBO. However, an endoscopy only reaches the duodenum and cannot retrieve samples of gut bacteria in the latter parts of the small intestine. Therefore, when looking for a doctor who tests for SIBO, be specific and ask if they utilize a SIBO breath test.

Hydrogen and methane gases are produced by bacteria in the small intestine that cross into the blood and then lungs. During a SIBO breath test, the patient will drink a sugar solution of glucose or lactulose which feeds the bacteria. The patient blows into a tube over the course of a few hours to measure the levels of hydrogen and methane gas expelled from the lungs.

The tricky part of SIBO testing is the doctor's interpretation of the patient's results. Some doctors may interpret a slight rise in breath gas levels as a positive marker of SIBO while others may require a significant rise in gas levels. Also, the preparation for the test requires the patient meet certain criteria for the test results to be considered valid. Ideally, patients should be off antibiotics and probiotics for a time as well as avoid certain bacteria-feeding foods.

X-ray

Most of you have likely had an x-ray or know of someone who has had an x-ray as they are common scans for various conditions, particularly for broken or fractured bones. The X-ray is an example of an imaging study that is an easy, quick way to take a snapshot of your insides.

Although an x-ray is useful for detecting broken bones, impacted bowels, or possibly a large tumor or mass, most gallstones will not show up on an x-ray, as most stones are composed primarily of cholesterol. X-ray also does not produce a detailed snapshot of the organs or the ducts. For this reason, your doctor or an emergency room physician may order an ultrasound as the first imaging study and skip the x-ray.

Gastric Emptying Study

The most common type of gastric emptying study is a scan that is done by a nuclear medicine physician to determine the rate at which food empties from your stomach into the small intestines. It utilizes x-ray and a small amount of radioactive material.

Before the scan, you'll eat something solid (usually scrambled eggs) and liquid, where one or both contain a small amount of tasteless radioactive material. The radioactive substance allows the scan to follow the food through the upper digestive system.

Once you have finished your meal, you will lie on or stand against a table while a special x-ray camera takes pictures. Over the course of three to five hours, the camera will take four to six scans lasting about a minute each. The rate at which the radioactivity leaves the stomach reflects the rate at which food is emptying from the stomach.

A below-normal emptying rate may indicate gastric outlet obstruction or gastroparesis. Above-normal emptying can cause diarrhea.

Upper and Lower GI Series

Upper and lower GI series use x-rays and barium, a chalky liquid, to examine the upper GI tract (esophagus, stomach, and first part of the small intestine) and lower GI tract (large intestine).

For an Upper GI, you will first drink the barium. You will then lay against an inverted table where a fluoroscope machine transmits images to a video monitor. The barium makes the pictures more visible as it passes through the digestive tract, from the esophagus then to the stomach, and finish at the duodenum.

This upper GI test is used to diagnose conditions like hiatal hernias, ulcers, tumors, esophageal varices, and obstruction or narrowing of the upper GI tract.

Lower GI tests or barium enemas are used to examine the large intestine and the rectum. For this test, barium or an iodine-containing liquid is introduced gradually into the colon through a tube inserted into the rectum. As the barium passes through the lower intestines, it fills the colon, allowing the radiologist to see growths or polyps and areas that are narrowed. The fluoroscope machine is held over the part of the body being examined and transmits continuous images to the video monitor.

The lower GI test is used to detect colon polyps, tumors, diverticular disease, gastroenteritis, strictures or sites of narrowing and obstruction, ulcerative colitis or Crohn's disease, and other causes of abdominal pain or blood, mucus, or pus in the stool

Ultrasound

Ultrasound is an imaging method that uses high-frequency sound waves to produce images of the inner workings of your organs and other structures within your body. If you are a woman who has been pregnant, you have most likely experienced an ultrasound to track the growth and health of your baby.

Ultrasound can show biliary or pancreatic duct stones and ductal changes. It can measure the size of the liver, pancreas, and ducts as well as show tumors and cysts. Ultrasound may also be used to view potential masses or other abnormalities of the stomach and intestines.

An external ultrasound does not produce a good snapshot of the pancreas as it sits behind the stomach, and is not a good tool for showing other organs, blood vessels, or tissue in detail. If your ultrasound is normal or your doctor or the radiologist finds something needing a better visual, he or she will likely order a CT scan or MRI as the next step. Most insurance companies require a series of tests before they will approve payment for costlier or invasive imaging studies.

CT Scan

A CT (Computed Tomography) scan combines x-ray with computerized technology to produce highly detailed images of organs, blood vessels, and tissues. Sometimes an iodine or barium based contrast agent, also known as a dye, will be administered either orally, rectally or via injection. The contrast will produce an enhanced visual of specific organs, blood vessels and/or tissues. Some people, especially those with kidney disease, cannot tolerate the contrast agent.

Although contrast is often preferred, it isn't necessarily needed to capture a visual. CT scans are rather quick and easy with few restrictions, unlike MRI. However, CT scans carry the most radiation risk of all imaging methods. According to Consumer Reports, "CT scans emit a powerful dose of radiation, in some cases equivalent to about 200 chest X-rays, or the amount most people would be exposed to from natural sources over seven years."

Every time I landed in an emergency room, the attending physician would order a CT scan. I didn't see this as a problem at the beginning of my journey, but am now very concerned about the amount of radiation exposure I have endured throughout my illness. I have had over a dozen CT scans. Most were not necessary. I did not know any better.

Today, if I am in the emergency room or hospital, I refuse CT scans unless it is a life or death situation. I say this not to scare you but to inform you. A CT scan at the beginning of your postcholecystectomy diagnostic journey may be necessary in revealing a glaring condition that needs to be addressed. Beyond that, I'd ask if there is an alternative imaging study the doctor can recommend.

MRI/MRCP

MRI (Magnetic Resonance Imaging) uses strong magnets and radio waves instead of radiation to create images of the digestive organs. It is not as detailed as a CT scan but is more detailed than an ultrasound. Some people who have implantable devices cannot get an MRI; and you must remain motionless for long periods of time. For postcholecystectomy syndrome, your doctor will likely order an MRCP (magnetic resonance cholangiopancreatography) rather than a standard MRI.

An MRCP is basically the same thing as an MRI, but it specifically evaluates the liver, gallbladder, bile duct, pancreas, and pancreatic duct for disease. Frequently, a contrast called gadolinium is used. It is a rare-earth mineral and is less likely to cause an allergic reaction compared to the iodinated contrast agents used in CT scanning. I never had a problem with it, but did know a woman with Lyme disease who had difficulty detoxifying heavy metals and was sick with weird symptoms for a few months after receiving gadolinium.

HIDA Scan

A HIDA scan, also known as a cholescintigraphy or hepatobiliary scintigraphy, is a test done by nuclear medicine physicians to diagnose bile duct obstructions, gallbladder disease, bile leaks, and issues with the sphincters.

You will likely be placed on your back for the test as it can take an hour or more. A radioactive tracer will be injected into a vein in your arm. The tracer travels through your bloodstream to your liver, and is then excreted by the bile-producing cells. The radioactive tracer travels with the bile from your liver into your gallbladder and through your bile ducts to your small intestine. Pretreatment of CCK hormone may improve the sensitivity for its detection. CCK is used to induce gallbladder contractions and is generally used to measure gallbladder functioning.

Emptying delayed by more than two hours or a prolonged half-time can help identify the sphincter of Oddi as a potential cause for your symptoms. However, it cannot differentiate between other conditions such as stenosis and dyskinesia. A HIDA scan, however, lacks adequate resolution to identify dilation and stricture. It also does not provide imaging of the pancreas, pancreatic duct, or functioning of the pancreatic sphincter.

Endoscopy and Colonoscopy

Endoscopy literally means "looking inside." A scope is put through the mouth, down the throat, into your esophagus, stomach, and duodenum until it reaches the entrance to the pancreatic and biliary ducts. This scope can take images and retrieve biopsy samples of tissue of the esophagus, stomach, and duodenum. Many upper gastrointestinal conditions like ulcers, celiac disease, bacterial infections, bile gastritis, hiatal hernia, and some cancers can be diagnosed via an endoscopy.

In addition, this procedure is used to rule out other conditions which could be causing your symptoms. An endoscopy procedure carries few complications. Most complications are related to the anesthesia. If you have any loose teeth, the tube could inadvertently force a tooth to come out. The tube can also irritate the throat and esophagus for several days.

A colonoscopy is an endoscopic evaluation of the large intestine or colon. Lower gastrointestinal issues like diverticulitis, polyps, Crohn's disease, ulcerative colitis, hemorrhoids, and some cancers can be diagnosed through colonoscopy. Like an endoscopy, it is also used to rule out other possible causes to your symptoms.

Patients often say the worst part of the colonoscopy is the prep the day before the procedure in which they must ingest a good amount of a laxative solution and as such spend much of their day and evening going to the bathroom. There are few risks. Like with an endoscopy, patients sometimes react to anesthesia. Other than that, a rare complication is bowel perforation.

For both the endoscopy and colonoscopy you will not be able to eat or drink after a certain time of the day or evening before the procedure. These are considered outpatient procedures, meaning you will be at the hospital or endoscopy center for part of a day and rarely need to be admitted overnight. Due to the sedation used during the procedure, you will not be able to drive for 24 hours. Most people do not remember their endoscopy or colonoscopy due to the sedation involved.

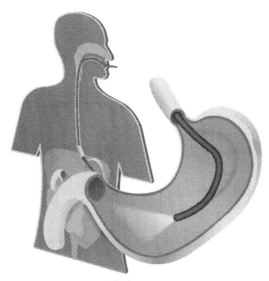

Endoscopy

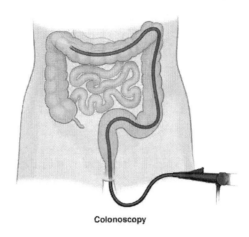

Colonoscopy

Endoscopic Ultrasound (EUS)

EUS is essentially an endoscopy scope with an ultrasound attachment on the end. The prep and after care is the same as an endoscopy. EUS can be used to diagnose diseases of the pancreas, bile duct, and gallbladder when other tests are inconclusive or conflicting. It can identify ductal changes like strictures and dilated ducts.

EUS is a good visual option in comparison to ERCP, which can cause acute pancreatitis. Another advantage of the EUS is a needle can be used to obtain a biopsy of the pancreas tissue to detect cellular abnormalities.

EUS is also used to evaluate known abnormalities, including lumps or lesions, which were detected at a prior endoscopy or were seen on an MRI or CT scan. EUS provides a detailed image of the lump or lesion, which can help your doctor determine its origin and help treatment decisions.

Endoscopic Retrograde Cholangiopancreatogram (ERCP)

ERCP is like an endoscopy and EUS as it uses a scope; and the prep and aftercare is similar. With an ERCP, a catheter is attached to the end of the scope. This catheter can inject a dye into the biliary and pancreatic ducts which will help to produce high quality x-rays of the ducts and organs. Other catheters and guidewires may be used to enter the ducts or measure the sphincter and ductal pressures (manometry). ERCP with sphincter of Oddi manometry is considered the "gold standard" in the diagnosis of SOD.

Diagnostic and Therapeutic Endoscopy defined sphincter hypertension as basal sphincter pressures above 40 mmHg and is considered manometric evidence of SOD. Theoretically, elevated sphincter pressures indicate the sphincter is prone to spasm, causing SOD symptoms. The higher the manometric reading, the worse the sphincter spasms.

Though it is the gold standard, even ERCP with manometry is not foolproof. Because of inconsistent results, manometry has become as controversial as SOD itself. One problem I found in researching manometry information is that it is not as standardized as it was a few decades ago.

This means that doctors have moved away from this method of diagnosing SOD; and there is no reliable data collection system gathering information on manometry results, symptoms, treatments, and outcomes. Subsequently, there is a lack of data sharing. Though studies show manometry does not contribute to acute pancreatitis, SOD doctors will perform a sphincterotomy, cutting the sphincter during ERCP, yet not bother to conduct manometry.

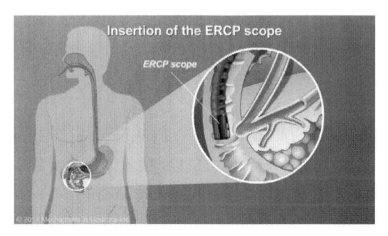

Insertion of the ERCP scope
ERCP scope

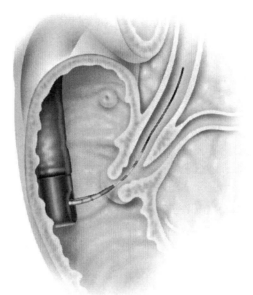

ERCP Scope with Guidewire in Bile Duct

Chapter 4 Postcholecystectomy Diet

Regardless of your postcholecystectomy symptoms or diagnosis, it is very important to follow certain dietary rules now that your body no longer has a gallbladder. The foods your body will have the most difficulty digesting are fats, even healthy fats. Bile, essential for digesting fats, is no longer concentrated or released in the manner it once was when you had a gallbladder.

You may have difficulty digesting proteins and high cholesterol foods like dairy and eggs as well. However, I don't recommend limiting your protein intake. Instead, space proteins out and eat them several times a day and not with a fatty meal. In fact, overall, frequent small meals will be easier on your digestive system after cholecystectomy. In other words, do not overeat!

Every time I dined at a restaurant I felt obligated to eat everything on my plate. Consequently, I'd suffer severe postcholecystectomy symptoms afterward. I'd head straight to bed, feeling like a beached whale afflicted with bloat, nausea, and pain. Like me and many others with no gallbladder, overeating can produce nightmare symptoms. It's not worth it! Eating reasonably-sized portions will put less strain on your liver and biliary system.

Practice eating half-portions and take the leftovers home to eat for another meal. At home or a dinner party, serve yourself up a smaller plate and don't go back for second helpings. The less food your digestive system must digest, the easier it will be for it to take its time, properly digesting in a symbiotic manner. And, always go easy on the fats.

This does not mean you should avoid all fats. Instead, be mindful of the amount of fat grams you ingest (Mayo Clinic recommends keeping it under 3 grams for cholecystectomy patients), especially saturated fats. As such, greasy and fried food may no longer be your friend. It is always wise to hold off on re-introducing fatty foods high in saturated fats shortly after your cholecystectomy. If you don't, you may experience pain, gas, or diarrhea.

Some of the worst offenders, besides fried foods, are cheese, fatty luncheon meats, sausages, hot dogs, fatty pieces of steak, dark meat portions of poultry, butter, and all oils except MCT oils.

LCT vs. MCT Fats

Postcholecystectomy patients will have a more difficult time digesting long-chain triglycerides (LCTs) as opposed to medium-chain triglycerides (MCTs). It is important to understand the difference between LCT and MCT fats and oils.

The fats in our food are composed almost entirely of LCTs. When we consume fats composed of LCTs they travel through the stomach and into the intestinal wall. It is in the intestines where most of fat digestion occurs. Pancreatic enzymes and bile are necessary for the digestion of LCT fats. LCTs are then reduced into individual long-chain fatty acids. These fatty acids are absorbed into the intestinal wall. Inside the intestinal wall, they are repackaged into bundles of fat and protein called lipoproteins. These lipoproteins are then sent into the bloodstream. As they circulate in the bloodstream, they release particles of fat.

This is the source of the fat that collects in our fat cells and the fat that collects in and clogs up artery walls. As the lipoproteins get smaller, they eventually go into the liver. In the liver, they are dismantled and used for energy or repackaged into new lipoproteins and again sent back into the bloodstream to disperse fat throughout the body.

MCT fats are processed differently. After eating a fat containing MCTs, such as coconut oil, it travels through the stomach and into the small intestine. However, since MCTs digest quickly, by the time they leave the stomach and enter the intestinal tract, they are already broken down into individual fatty acids. Therefore, they do not need pancreatic enzymes or bile for digestion.

Since MCTs are already reduced to fatty acids as they enter the small intestine, they are immediately absorbed into the portal vein and sent straight to the liver. In the liver, they are preferentially used as a source of fuel to produce energy. These fatty acids bypass the lipoprotein stage in the intestinal wall and in the liver. They do not circulate in the bloodstream to the degree that other fats do. Therefore, they do not supply the fat that collects in fat cells nor do they supply the fat that collects in artery walls.

The easy assimilation of MCTs by the body allows increased absorption of other nutrients. Studies show that MCTs enhance the absorption of minerals, particularly calcium and magnesium. They improve the absorption of some of the B vitamins, the fat-soluble vitamins (A, D, E, K, and beta-carotene), as well as amino acids. There is a reason MCTs exist in breast milk.

Therefore, as your bile output and consistency may be compromised as a person without a gallbladder, stick to MCT fats like coconut oil and palm kernel oil. Butter, whole milk, and cheese all contain MCT fat but they also may contain a high amount of LCT fat. Limit these. Otherwise "healthy fats" may not be so healthy. Foods touted as healthy fats like avocado, olive oil, nuts, and fatty fish may not be so healthy for a postcholecystectomy patient.

Keep in mind that although MCT oils are great alternatives for cooking and acquiring fat for energy, it is well-known that MCTs are not a good source of essential fatty acids. Therefore, if your diet is high in MCTs, you will want to supplement essential fatty acids like Omega 3 and 6, which will be discussed in Chapter 5.

Food Diary and Elimination Diet

If you are experiencing unexplained symptoms and suspect certain foods may be the culprit, I suggest starting a food and symptom diary. Food diaries are easy tools to identify trigger and safe foods. There is no hard rule of what this diary should look like, but a good food and symptom diary is broken down by daily time intervals like morning, mid-morning, noon, afternoon, evening, and late evening. You may keep notes in a notebook, on your computer, or in your phone.

In fact, there are a variety of free and affordable food diary apps you can download for your phone or tablet. Whatever form of a food diary you choose doesn't matter as long as you are diligent in recording everything you put in your mouth, i.e. food, beverages, supplements and medications; and the symptoms you feel throughout the day. This will help you identify what is safe and not safe to consume. Activities like exercise or meditation should also be included.

The food diary doesn't just isolate foods as they affect you. Absolutely anything you ingest is fair game for triggering postcholecystectomy symptoms. Seemingly innocent vitamins, minerals, herbal supplements, and medications can be triggers.

I have allergies and found if I ingested certain herbal teas like chamomile I'd get stomach cramps and headaches. This made sense because I have seasonal allergies and chamomile is an herb. In other words, if I was allergic to breathing in a plant, then of course my body would react to ingesting it.

Beverages could also be an issue. I would develop severe pain after drinking carbonated drinks like soda or seltzer. I tried changing soda brands and flavors, thinking it was the artificial flavorings, colorings or sweeteners of a particular brand. I soon discovered soda, even sparkling water, caused pain and concluded it was the carbonation, not the ingredients which caused the problem. My theory was the air from the carbonation got "stuck" in the ducts as the sphincters spasm open and shut (from my SOD), causing pressure and pain.

Deducing the origin of symptom triggers takes investigative work and patience. Some food reactions may be instant while others are delayed. You may experience a symptom from a food several hours after ingesting and confuse the reaction with a food you ate later. For this reason, I recommend starting your food diary with a strict food elimination plan then slowly reintroduce the foods and treats you like.

Don't eat the same thing two days in a row. Also, foods with multiple ingredients should be kept to a minimum. For example, I know many postcholecystectomy patients who react to mashed potatoes. The problem with mashed potatoes is there are several ingredients which could cause the problem, i.e. potatoes, milk, butter, seasonings, etc. If you had a plain potato and it didn't bother you, but mashed potatoes did, then undoubtedly you are sensitive to the dairy or the fat content of the added ingredients. Even a seemingly innocent seasoning could be to blame.

Most elimination diets are meant to identify allergies or food sensitivities. Postcholecystectomy triggers are not allergies per se, but having no gallbladder may lead to food sensitivities or intolerances especially if bile and pancreatic enzyme output is impeded. Most food elimination plans will recommend eliminating the most common food allergy/sensitivity offenders like dairy, nuts, soy, eggs, peanuts, gluten, etc.

The key is keeping it simple in the beginning to foods like rice, lean meat, vegetables, and some fruits. At the very least, eliminate the most commonly reported postcholecystectomy triggers. Some of these are:

Fried foods
Spicy foods
Fatty and oily foods
Coffee and anything with caffeine
Chocolate
Red meat and pork, even lean cuts
Alcohol
Some fruits especially acidic fruits
Difficult-to-digest raw vegetables

Track your symptoms and within a few days try to reintroduce foods one at a time. Have a good amount of the food so you can see if it causes symptoms. Continue to reintroduce foods one at a time every few days. If a food doesn't make your symptoms flare, keep that food in your diet. Anything that causes a flare up should be eliminated. After a week or two, try adding it back again. If it continues causes a flare up, eliminate it for good from your diet.

Juicing and Blending

Many postcholecystectomy patients report feeling better when they eat a juiced or blended diet for one or for all meals. You may want to stick to juicing and blending during your food elimination stage. Juicing and blending are different but similar. Both make it easier for your body to absorb nutrients as they are in the form of micronutrients. A juiced vegetable may take less than 30 minutes to digest while its raw whole counterpart could take 6 hours or more.

Juicing vegetables and fruits with a juicer (not to be confused with an extractor) squeezes juice from the food. None of the fibers or proteins are included in the juice extract and nutrients are more easily and quickly absorbed.

Blending or extracting (think Ninja or Vitamix appliance) emulsifies the vegetable or fruit, leaving the juice and fibers intact. For some people, this can be an issue as it is very high in fiber. A high fiber diet is contraindicated for people with certain intestinal conditions and those with post-gallbladder diarrhea. If you are someone who does better with extra fiber, or experiences constipation, then this may be the way to go. However, for those who are sensitive to high fiber diets, you may want to stick with juicing.

I recommend homemade blended smoothies before drinking preservative- and artificial ingredient-laden drinks like Ensure or Muscle Milk. You can make smoothies with any kind of pure protein powder. Whey is a popular protein powder. I buy undenatured raw organic whey made from the milk of grass fed cows. It is purer and less processed than standard whey proteins.

Processed whey can literally be junk for your digestive system as it is usually made from the milk of cows fed high grain diets and given antibiotics and hormones. Also, high processed whey is known to be excitotoxic due to its high glutamate content. For this reason, people with nervous system issues should steer clear of processed whey.

Rice, pea or hemp protein powder are good choices as well but may be gritty. The only protein I absolutely do not recommend is soy protein, as it can be inflammatory. Anytime I ingest soy in any form, my joints and tendons ache.

Once you have selected a protein powder, put a few scoops in a blender and add vegetables and fruits and/or their juice/extract, yogurt or kefir (a yogurt drink) if you want, ice, coconut water, and a healthy fat like coconut oil (keep to less than a teaspoon). It isn't fun living on a liquid diet, but can be useful during severe flare ups as a meal replacement. There are also good medical food replacement powders you can purchase. They are advertised as meal replacements and some as leaky gut supplements.

Liver-Healing Vegetables and Fruits

The juice of certain vegetables can do wonders for the liver and biliary system. Beets, apples, and ginger all support bile formation. Beets are probably the best vegetable for your liver as they are a high-antioxidant vegetable that contain important substances like betaine, betalains, fiber, iron, betacyanin, folate, and betanin.

Pectin, which is a fiber found in beets, can also help clean the toxins that have been removed from the liver, allowing them to be flushed out of the system instead of reabsorbed by the body. Betaine is the substance that encourages the liver cells to get rid of toxins. Additionally, betaine acts to defend the liver and bile ducts, which are important if the liver is to function properly. This substance is also said to decrease the risk of coronary and cerebral artery disease.

Additionally, beets have been linked to healing the liver, decreasing homocysteine levels (which could reduce the risk of heart disease, Alzheimer's and stroke), an improvement in stomach acid production, prevention of the formation of free-radicals in LDL (the bad cholesterol), and the prevention of lung, liver, skin, spleen, and colon cancer. Though these health benefits are not directly linked to the detoxification of the liver, they allow the body to work more efficiently. Because the systems of the body are all intertwined and rely upon one another to work properly, this indirectly affects the ability of the liver to rid itself of toxins and continue to work at an optimal level.

Apples contain malic acid which helps to open the bile ducts that run through your liver and reportedly soften and release gallstones. Apples are also high in pectin.

Ginger is reported to increase gut motility and bile production. You can add ginger to food dishes or eat it raw. I prefer to juice ginger and drink a small amount of the extract. The extract can also be added to juiced fruits and vegetables. Be careful, though, as ginger is spicy and pungent. You only need a small amount.

Lemon is purported to benefit the liver as well. The high citrate content in lemon increases the liver's ability to remove toxins. In addition, lemon contains a bioflavonoid called hesperidin, which protects the liver from damage, assists with digestion in the stomach (enhancing the effect of stomach acid), and inhibits fat synthesis, which is beneficial for fatty liver disease.

Other foods reported to protect the liver and increase bile production are bitter foods such as dandelion and mustard greens, radishes, artichokes, fruits high in vitamin c, and cruciferous vegetables such as broccoli, cauliflower, and cabbage.

Good Diet Habits

I recommend trying your best to eat organic and non-processed foods. Ideally, shop in the outer aisles of the grocery store. I particularly steer clear of GMO foods, which are engineered to withstand large applications of Roundup, a toxic fertilizer. GMO foods aren't the same foods our ancestors ate, which could mean they are harder to digest. Typically, products free of GMOs will state on their labels "GMO free" or "No GMOs".

I also advocate consuming only antibiotic free meat. The antibiotics injected into animals are often powerful and can be neurotoxic. Quite often the meat industry uses fluoroquinolone antibiotics which were invented to kill Anthrax! These antibiotics end up in our bodies, disrupting our precious microbiome bacteria environment. Your liver will love you for keeping your diet clean as it won't have to work overtime to detoxify foods containing pesticides, preservatives, artificial flavorings and coloring and other toxins.

The liver experiences a great deal of strain acclimating to digesting without a gallbladder. When we flood our bodies with toxic substances, our liver, pancreas, and intestines must work extra hard to remove them from the body. Ideally, bile acts as a detergent to break down fats and carry toxins out of the body. However, as discussed, bile consistency isn't the same after cholecystectomy.

Keep in mind, not all bile is eliminated through our stools, but instead, is reabsorbed by the intestine and sent back to the liver. These toxins can end up back in the liver where it joins more toxins accumulated from the present. The more work the liver must do the more stress to the biliary system, pancreas and possibly the sphincters. Stay away from high fructose corn syrup too as it is the leading contributor to fatty liver disease.

As discussed previously, do not overeat. Gluttony is not your friend after cholecystectomy. The more food and variety of foods you ingest in one sitting, the more strain you put on your liver and biliary system. Instead, eat frequent small meals. Practice chewing your food for a count of 20-30 chews depending on the food's consistency. Eat half portions for breakfast, lunch, and dinner and add healthy snacks at mid-morning and late afternoon. It is not advised to eat or snack after dinner. The fasting period between dinner and breakfast will aid your digestive system to recover and rejuvenate for optimal digestion the next day.

Specific Diets

Some postcholecystectomy patients report benefiting from specific diets, the most common being anything low-fat. I have several low-fat cookbooks on my computer tablet, so meals don't get boring and I don't feel deprived. You can find an abundance of low-fat diet cookbooks online for free, as apps, and in the form of books.

I don't think anyone with postcholecystectomy symptoms can go wrong with a low-fat diet. Some find it helpful to count fat grams and keep it under a certain amount as determined by their food diary. Therefore, I won't tell you the exact number of fat grams you need to focus on as everyone is different. Here is an example of low-fat food options:

White meat chicken or turkey
Pork tenderloin or other lean pork portion (although some people have issues with pork)
Low-fat fish options, i.e. cod, flounder, sole, white meat tuna, halibut, and haddock
Shellfish
Any bread labeled low-fat
Saltine crackers or other low-fat crackers
Fruits and vegetables--any and all you can tolerate except avocado
Low-fat or fat free yogurt, milk, cheese, etc.
Beans or bean products

I don't recommend nuts, seeds, or peanuts as they are extremely high in fat and difficult to digest. However, some nut flours aren't too high in fat their content and retain the nut's protein. Read labels to discern fat grams.

Along with a low-fat diet, my gastroenterologist and dietician recommended I adopt the FODMAP diet. It is usually reserved for irritable bowel syndrome and SIBO, but some with other postcholecystectomy conditions find it helpful. FODMAP stands for Fermentable Oligosaccharides, Disaccharides, Monosaccharides and Polyols. These foods contain difficult-to-digest sugars and fibers that can cause bowel problems like excess gas, painful bloating, and constipation or diarrhea.

You can perform an Internet search for "FODMAP" and find many different websites on this topic along with lists of which foods to avoid and which are safe foods. As of this writing, I found that dietician Kate Scarlata's website provided the most comprehensive information on the FODMAP diet. Examples of common foods to avoid are wheat, onion, garlic, beans, apples, lactose-containing dairy, and high fructose sweeteners.

Another diet strategy many people with postcholecystectomy syndrome employ is to go gluten free. Gluten is not only linked to celiac disease, but also "leaky gut", a condition where the lining of the small intestine is damaged.

Gluten-free is a big craze now, but I am yet to meet anyone whose postcholecystectomy symptoms were completely relieved from a gluten free diet. Some people do report feeling better having gone gluten-free but it is likely these people had celiac disease or a gluten sensitivity. Going gluten-free is not a panacea for curing your postcholecystectomy symptoms. However, for some people, a gluten-free diet will enable a patient to eat better, quality foods, which could help their symptoms.

One thing to consider and be leery of is there are a lot of gluten-free items with nasty ingredients that could trigger symptoms. When my postcholecystectomy symptoms were at their worst, I went gluten-free for a whole year. I was strict about it and felt no better or worse. I personally do not believe gluten is entirely evil, but I do try to limit the amount of gluten I eat in a week.

If I do want to avoid gluten, I focus more on eating clean, whole food options like lean organic proteins, vegetables, and fruits. There is certainly no harm in trying a gluten-free lifestyle. Just stick with healthy food choices and not gluten-free items loaded with sugar, fat, and ingredients you can't pronounce.

Food Combining

With postcholecystectomy syndrome, you will want to make digestion as easy a process as possible. Food combining can accomplish this as eating some food groups together can be a disaster for your digestive system. Food combining enthusiasts recommend never eating a heavy protein with a heavy carbohydrate or starch. In other words, eating meat and a potato together is a no-no. The same goes for meat with pasta or bread. Instead, eat meats, beans, or tofu with a non-starchy vegetable. Pair heavy carbohydrates with a non-starchy vegetable.

As for fruit, eat fruit alone, on an empty stomach. When fruits are eaten alone, your stomach can more easily process all the nutrients, fiber and sugars contained in the fruit.

Avoid large amounts of fat with protein combined with a carbohydrate because it slows digestion. This is one of the reasons pizza is a postcholecystectomy nightmare food. Pizza has all the big offenders: heavy fatty protein (cheese) and a heavy carbohydrate, high in FODMAPs (wheat pizza dough). The tomato sauce is likely ok unless it has a high amount of onions and garlic which are high in FODMAPs, or you are sensitive to the acidity in tomatoes. I love pizza, but it always brought on pain and indigestion.

Salad dressings and sandwich spreads are notoriously high in fat content. Mayonnaise, oil and vinegar, ranch, and other dressings are super high in fat. Alternatively, use mustard or a low-fat dressing on a sandwich. Avoid prepared sandwich salads like chicken salad and tuna. They are usually loaded with mayonnaise. Dress your salads with squeezed lemon and salad dressings labeled "low-fat". When dining out, ask your server to recommend a low-fat salad dressing option.

Final Word on Diet

In closing, I think it is fitting I mention that one of my worst triggers was going too long without eating. Yes, not eating triggered postcholecystectomy symptoms. I thought I was alone with this issue until I met others who experienced the same thing. It was as if the stress of being hungry caused pain. Also, our bodies will automatically signal when to release bile at certain times of the day. Therefore, bile could be released without food added to the mix. For some people, this causes bile acid diarrhea.

Again, don't eat fast. Instead, chew your food thoroughly and take your time. This will benefit your entire digestive tract and organs so they don't have to work as hard. Your digestive system starts in your mouth where enzymes are released to start the digestion process. Taking the time to allow these enzymes to mix with your food is essential for proper and thorough digestion.

Chapter 5: Natural Treatments

Natural treatments will depend on your postcholecystectomy symptoms and condition. What may work for one condition may hinder another. It's also important to keep in mind that with almost every "remedy" you must give it some time to see if it will help you. Doing anything once or twice and giving up on it is not what this is all about. Relief will not magically happen overnight. Try different things and give each treatment some time to see if it will work. Be patient.

Before embarking on your natural remedy journey, I recommend you invest in a consult or two with one or more of the following natural health practitioners:

Naturopathic Doctor—Treats patients using natural therapies such as physical manipulation, clinical nutrition, herbal medicine, homeopathy, counseling, acupuncture, and hydrotherapy. They choose treatments based on the individual patient, not based on the generality of symptoms. For some who prefer only a natural treatment route, they have made a naturopathic doctor their primary care physician.

Functional Medicine Doctor or Practitioner—Addresses the underlying causes of disease, engaging both patient and practitioner in a therapeutic partnership and individualized treatment plan. These practitioners address the whole person, not just an isolated set of symptoms, moving away from the traditional disease-centered focus of medical practice to a more patient-centered approach. These practitioners can be a medical doctor, nurse practitioner, pharmacist, chiropractor, or other licensed health professional who completed specialized training in this area of practice.

Chiropractor—Focuses on the diagnosis and treatment of neuromuscular disorders, with an emphasis on treatment through manual adjustment and/or manipulation of the spine. Today, many chiropractors are cross-trained in the same complimentary therapies naturopathic and functional medicine doctors practice.

<u>Holistic Health Counselors and Nutritionists, Homeopaths, and Herbalists</u>—Treat the whole person in the same manner as a naturopath or functional medicine practitioner but with less schooling. Relies mostly on homeopathic medicine, diet, herbs, and other natural remedies to treat the patient.

Most of these practitioners can assess your current health status through traditional examinations and bloodwork, order alternative diagnostic testing, and "prescribe" some of the natural remedies listed in this chapter. Seeking a consult with a natural health practitioner is likely a better option rather than going rogue on your own, trialing various supplements.

Share the content of this chapter with your natural health practitioner or physician as they may think one or more of these natural remedies could benefit you.

But First a Word on Liver Flushes and Detoxes

If you search the Internet for gallbladder or postcholecystectomy treatments, you will find many sites touting gallbladder or liver flushes and detoxes. I am here to tell you, "BEWARE!" These flushes are commonly touted to clean out the gallbladder or liver and rid the body of multiple gallstones, even "re-setting" the liver.

Most liver flushes are harsh and put a great deal of stress on the liver and biliary system. In some instances, they can be beneficial, i.e. if you still get stones. However, steer clear, as it could worsen the condition by putting more strain on the already strained organs and ducts.

Most liver flushes call for a combination of Epsom salts, olive oil, and lemon sometimes preceded by ingestion of an apple. I tried this flush once and ended up with a stomach ache that lingered for months. I am not kidding—months! I think it was the Epsom salts. Epsom salts, when ingested, is a harsh laxative made of magnesium salts. Although magnesium in small quantities can be beneficial, the concentration of it in Epsom salts is massive and can burden your entire digestive system.

Instead of a liver flush touted on the Internet, I recommend sticking to another natural treatment.

Supplements

Did you ever walk into a health food store and feel overwhelmed with the variety of supplement options in front of you? There are literally thousands of supplements purported to aid digestive woes and improve digestion. Attempting to decipher which supplement will help your postcholecystectomy symptoms will be difficult unless under the care of a natural health practitioner.

For informational purposes, the following supplements described herein have been recommended by other postcholecystectomy patients, personally trialed by me, or heavily researched for postcholecystectomy symptoms. Some are benign and could be trialed on your own. However, with any supplement, talk to your primary care physician to ensure none are contraindicated for your health conditions or medications you are taking.

Essential Fatty Acids

Fatty acids are important for all systems of the body to function normally, including your skin, respiratory system, circulatory system, brain, and organs. There are two fatty acids, termed essential fatty acids (EFA) that your body does not produce on its own. EFAs must be ingested through oils, i.e. olive, flax seed, and fish. The two primary EFAs are known as linoleic acid (omega-6) and alpha-linolenic acid (omega-3).

These EFAs are necessary for the following processes:

Formation of healthy cell membranes
Proper development and functioning of the brain and nervous system
Proper thyroid and adrenal activity
Hormone production

Regulation of blood pressure, liver function, immune and inflammatory responses
Regulation of blood clotting
Crucial for the transport and breakdown of cholesterol
Support healthy skin and hair
Vision
Nervous system and brain function

As discussed previously, when your gallbladder is no longer intact, bile production and bile's consistency changes, making it difficult for some patients to properly digest fats. Therefore, the essential fatty acids we need for healthy functioning are compromised as they may not be converted or absorbed. Dr. Mercola, of the popular Mercola website, used a great analogy, "Trying to digest fat without bile is like trying to wash greasy dishes without soap--it doesn't work very well." If your gallbladder is removed, then you may benefit with supplementing these fatty acids.

Although Omega 6 and Omega 3 EFAs are both equally essential, the amount of each supplement necessary for therapeutic purposes varies. It isn't as easy as popping a few pills. The ratio of Omega 6 and Omega 3 is important as a higher ratio of Omega 3 is associated with reducing disease, inflammation, and improving overall bodily and immune functions.

I learned accidentally how important an Omega 3 supplement was. Since my gallbladder removal, I suffered from very dry eyes. I used to wear contact lenses all the time, but after my cholecystectomy, contacts felt like shards of glass stuck to my eyes. My ophthalmologist recommended I take 1200mg of an Omega 3 supplement every day. To balance things out, I took one combo supplement of Omega 3, 6 and 9, but always twice as much Omega 3 as Omega 6. Believe it or not, my eyes weren't as dry anymore, and I started wearing contacts on occasion. I'm not sure if it's helping any other part of my body, but not having dry, red eyes is a bonus!

There are many different types of Omega 3 and 6 supplements available. Most are in the form of fish or krill oil. I take a pharmaceutical grade Omega 3 supplement that does not produce a nasty fish aftertaste. Some supplements, especially the cheaper versions, can produce fishy burps. Therefore, look for a supplement that advertises "no fish aftertaste."

Bile Acids

For digestive symptoms like indigestion, gas, constipation and bloating, supplementing with bile acids may help remedy your woes. You can find bile salts online or in a health food store. A natural health practitioner may carry them as well and be helpful in guiding you to a correct dosage. The dosage of bile salts will depend on the brand, the type of bile salt, and the milligram content of the supplement.

You may need to adjust the amount of bile salts to your own comfort level as too much can lead to diarrhea. Bile salts are best taken with a meal, as they provide the acids needed to digest your food. Strict vegetarians and vegans will not be able to take bile salts as they are generally made from animal bile.

Digestive Enzymes

Your digestive system breaks down the nutrients you consume in food, converting them into small molecules that your cells, tissues, and organs use as fuel and for hundreds of metabolic functions. It takes hours to complete this complex process, which results in simple sugars, fatty acids, glycerol (a sugar alcohol) and amino acids. After you break food into small pieces by chewing it, specialized enzymes made in different parts of your digestive tract act on it to finalize the process.

The three most important enzymes are amylase, protease, and lipase. Amylase is a digestive enzyme that acts on starch in food, breaking it down into smaller carbohydrate molecules. First, salivary glands in your mouth make salivary amylase, which begins the digestive process by breaking down starch when you chew your food, converting it into maltose, a smaller carbohydrate. Second, pancreatic amylase completes digestion of carbohydrates, producing glucose, a simple sugar necessary for energy that is absorbed into your blood and carried throughout your body.

Protease is any enzyme that breaks down protein into its building blocks, amino acids. Your digestive tract produces a number of these enzymes, but the three main proteases are pepsin, trypsin, and chymotrypsin. Special cells in your stomach produce pepsin, which breaks chemical bonds in proteins, producing smaller molecules called peptides. Your pancreas makes protease (trypsin and chymotrypsin), which completes protein digestion, producing simple amino acids that are absorbed into your circulation.

Lipase is an enzyme that breaks down dietary fats into smaller molecules called fatty acids and glycerol. A small amount of lipase, called gastric lipase, is made by cells in your stomach. The main source of lipase in your digestive tract is your pancreas, which makes pancreatic lipase that acts in your small intestine. First, bile made in your liver and released into your intestine converts dietary fat into small fatty globules. Pancreatic lipase acts on these fat globules, converting them into fatty acids and glycerol.

Although amylase, protease, and lipase are the three main enzymes your body uses to digest food, many other specialized enzymes also help in the process. Cells that line your intestines make enzymes called maltase, sucrase, and lactase, each able to convert a specific type of sugar into glucose. Similarly, special cells in your stomach secrete two other enzymes—renin and gelatinase. Renin acts on proteins in milk, converting them into smaller molecules called peptides, which are then fully digested by pepsin. Gelatinase digests gelatin and collagen, two large proteins in meat, into moderately-sized compounds whose digestion is then completed by pepsin, trypsin, and chymotrypsin, producing amino acids.

There are many reasons digestive enzymes could help your postcholecystectomy symptoms. If your bile has changed in consistency, i.e. thick bile, or you have sphincter of Oddi dysfunction, your pancreas may not be secreting the proper amount of enzymes required to get the job done. In one study, 46% of patients who had pancreatitis had thick or viscous bile, indicating that thick bile will affect the function of the pancreas.

You can supplement with over the counter or prescription (discussed in next chapter) digestive enzymes. Choosing an over the counter enzyme can be overwhelming as there are hundreds of enzyme complexes available. Generally, for postcholecystectomy syndrome, you want a supplement high in lipase. Here are some general guidelines:

Protease: A minimum of 33,000 HUT should be adequate for most meals. (Remember, you can always take a second or third capsule for protein meals that require it.)
Acid stable protease: 1,000 SAPU would be great. Most formulas have none.
Lipase: 5,000 LU is adequate.
Amylase: Look for 12,000 SKB.
Lactase: 1,500 LACU is the minimum with 2,000 or even 2,500 being better.

Look for a variety of other enzyme ingredients such as malt diastase, invertase, glucoamylase, cellulase, and hemicellulase. However, you don't want a supplement overrun with a bunch of ingredients. Amylase, protease, and lipase should be the primary ingredients.

Herbs

I typically do not recommend herbs for postcholescystectomy syndrome, not because herbs can't help, but some can worsen symptoms depending on the patient. The most popular herbs increase bile flow which can spell disaster if you have a blockage from a stone or biliary sludge. In addition, drug-induced liver injury has been linked to herbs. Therefore, I recommend seeking the guidance of a natural health practitioner to determine which herb or supplement is best for your individual symptoms.

That being said, here are the most common herbs used by postcholecystectomy patients:

Bitters—a concoction of herbs that will stimulate the flow of bile in the gall bladder, assisting in the digestion of fats. Dandelion root or leaf is a classic bitter liver tonic herb. Along with Oregon grape root bark, gentian root, and wormwood leaves, dandelion stimulates digestion, stimulates the liver to produce more bile.

Artichoke leaf extract—a potent "cholagogic" herb, which stimulates the production and secretion of bile by the gall bladder. This is due to the artichoke's cinarin content. Cinarin is a phytochemical that gives artichokes their semi-sweet taste.

Milk Thistle—protects liver cells by coating them with phytochemicals. These chemicals heal damaged liver cells and protect healthy cells from becoming damaged.

Oregon grape root—often used for acne, due to its anti-bacterial, anti-inflammatory properties. It also has bile-stimulating properties.

Gentian root extract—a natural fungicide and immune booster that possesses anti-inflammatory properties. Its bitter nature stimulates the secretion of both gastric juices and bile.

Valerian—an herb with natural muscle relaxant/antispasmodic qualities. I prefer valerian tea or valerian that is "standardized" in a gel cap. Valerian can make you drowsy, which is great if you are taking it at night, but not so great during the day. I have seen some extended release versions of valerian which may work better and reduce drowsiness as the herb is slowly absorbed by the body over a longer period.

Turmeric

Turmeric is a root and an ingredient in curry dishes. Turmeric is touted for its antioxidant and anti-inflammatory properties. It is purported to protect the liver and reduce cholesterol levels. It has been observed that turmeric reduced inflammation, fibrosis (scarring and thickening of tissue) and reduced bile duct obstruction in cholangitis patients.

Turmeric can be ingested by grating or juicing the fresh root. Additionally, there are many turmeric supplements available. A standardized version or one advertised as high in curcumin is best as it contains the highest levels of curcumin, the substance giving turmeric its healing qualities.

Choline

Choline is an essential nutrient that aides in the absorption of fat and cholesterol and helps your liver create lipoproteins, which are involved in many important cellular functions throughout your body. According to an article written by Dr. Mary Ackerley, a homeopathic physician, choline supplementation after gallbladder removal surgery helps support the natural digestion of dietary fats and can work well in combination with bile salts to help prevent excessive gas and bloating.

Betaine

Betaine (not to be confused with Betaine HCL) is another nutrient that helps your body breakdown and absorb fats, as described previously about beets. This nutrient helps maintain your metabolism and limits some of the side effects, such as bloating, gas, and diarrhea, following surgery. You can typically find betaine in capsule or powder form. Limit the recommended dose to 1-2 grams a day.

Lecithin

Lecithin is a supplement that supports digestive function following gallbladder removal. Research suggests that this substance keeps cholesterol from solidifying in your body and helps support your digestion of fats. You can get lecithin by eating foods such as oatmeal, eggs, and peanuts. Alternatively, you can take 500 to 1,000 milligrams daily in the form of a supplement or powder.

Soluble Fiber

Soluble fiber may benefit patients experiencing bile diarrhea or bile reflux. If we don't eat enough soluble fiber, our bile, instead of being ushered out of the body and then replaced with fresh bile produced by the liver, is repeatedly recirculated in our system. In the process, it becomes more concentrated with toxins, which, in turn, can lead to all sorts of inflammatory diseases such as gallbladder disease, intestinal inflammation, and even skin conditions like acne, eczema, and psoriasis.

Soluble fiber is unable to cross the intestinal barrier. Any substance that is bound to this fiber will likewise be unable to cross the intestinal barrier. Therefore, the liver will not receive back that bile from the gastro-intestinal tract. Theoretically, that means the liver will have to make new bile.

Examples of soluble fiber are beans, oats and other grains, certain fruits (apricots, grapefruit, mangoes, and oranges), flax seeds, and vegetables. There is also a wide range of fiber supplements you can purchase like methylcellulose, acacia, psyllium husk, calcium polycarbophil, wheat dextrose, or calcium polycarbophil.

Magnesium

Postcholecystectomy patients have reported that supplementing with magnesium helped them, probably due to its natural antispasmodic qualities. Oral magnesium is fine. but not if you have an issue with loose stools as magnesium is a natural laxative. If you tend to get constipated, then magnesium may not only help your symptoms but also get you going, if you know what I mean.

Alternatives to ingesting magnesium are magnesium oil and Epsom salt baths. Magnesium oil can be applied anywhere on the skin. I don't know how effective it is topically as studies are inconclusive. I used it topically for leg cramps, and it worked great. Same goes for Epsom salt baths. A bath with a ¼ to ½ cup of Epsom salts is supposed to provide a good amount of magnesium through the skin.

There are also natural health practitioners and functional medicine practitioners who offer magnesium injections. One woman I met in an online support group, who was suffering from postcholecystectomy pain, raved how magnesium injections significantly reduced her pain spasms.

Fat-Soluble Vitamins

Since bile helps your body absorb fat-soluble vitamins such as vitamins A, D, E and K, you may need to supplement some or all of these to reach optimal levels. Your body needs fat to absorb these vitamins as they dissolve in fat and can be stored in your liver and fat tissue until needed. Therefore, if you are following a strict, low-fat diet, your body won't have the adequate fat needed to absorb these nutrients.

Fat-soluble vitamins are essential for mineral absorption, strong bones and muscles, healthy eyes, protecting the body from free radicals, and blood clotting. Your doctor should order bloodwork measuring the levels of these vitamins to determine if you need to supplement. Since fat-soluble vitamins are stored in the liver and fat tissue, taking more than you need can lead to toxic levels.

Because some postcholecystectomy patients may be deficient in fat-soluble vitamins, it is advised to not ingest mineral oil (a common remedy for constipation) as it can interfere with your body's absorption of fat-soluble vitamins.

Probiotics

Our gut bacteria are like little mini engines controlling hormones, enzymes, metabolism, nervous system, digestion, and more. Probiotics boost our body's supply of good bacteria and are believed to crowd out bad bacteria. I can't say if probiotics ever helped my symptoms as I only took them to heal my gut after antibiotics. For that purpose, they were useful.

Studies are inconclusive regarding the efficacy of probiotics on liver diseases. Some studies have shown probiotics benefited fatty liver disease and biliary cholangitis infections, while others showed no positive effect. However, probiotics have been shown in numerous studies to improve IBS conditions and colonic infections.

I have tried numerous probiotics and found VSL 3 (http://www.vsl3.com) to be the best for me. It is the most studied probiotic and can be ordered online or prescribed by a doctor. The downside is that it is expensive, which seems to be the case for anything good for our health. Be careful taking probiotics as too much could cause small intestinal bacterial overgrowth.

Betaine HCL with Pepsin

This supplement is not to be confused with betaine without the HCL component. I take a betaine HCL (hydrochloride) supplement that includes pepsin to balance stomach acid, especially when I am experiencing bile reflux. Betaine HCL is a natural acid that promotes an acidic environment in the stomach. Pepsin is necessary for digesting proteins.

Contrary to popular belief, we need stomach acid for proper digestion, particularly protein digestion, and nutrient absorption. Stomach acid is also necessary for keeping bacteria in check and pathogens out. Unfortunately, doctors are quick to prescribe acid reducing medications like proton pump inhibitors (PPIs) and antacids, assuming a patient has too much stomach acid. Many patients actually suffer from other conditions like bile reflux, hiatal hernia, faulty esophageal or stomach sphincters, or low stomach acid. Studies show that stomach acid levels decrease with age and the symptoms of low stomach acid mimic those of excessive stomach acid and acid reflux.

Researchers are now finding a whole host of problems in people taking acid reducing medications on a long-term basis, including osteoporosis, mineral deficiencies, and dementia. Therefore, doctors should not prescribe PPIs or acid-reducing medications unless they have tested the patient's stomach ph. Unfortunately, ph testing is rarely performed on patients complaining of acid-reflux or gastritis (stomach inflammation) symptoms.

Betaine HCL helps if you have low stomach acid or there is bile present in the stomach, as bile acid is actually not an acid, but is closer to the neutral or basic end of the ph scale. Essentially, too much bile in the stomach will neutralize stomach acid. Therefore, if you are like me and experience bile reflux after cholecystectomy, bile ending up in the stomach will reduce the efficacy of your stomach's acid.

There are many betaine HCL supplements, some containing bitters or other added ingredients. I stick to a simple betaine HCL with pepsin formula with no added herbs. The patient should try taking one before a meal. If there is too much of a burning sensation, you likely do not need this supplement or your stomach needs to get used to the supplement. You can play around with the dose to see how much you need based on the level of burning in your stomach. Don't worry, though, most patients report this burning is neither uncomfortable or painful.

Lifestyle and Alternative Therapies

For some postcholecystectomy patients, the answer to their suffering may not be in a supplement or a pill bottle. Instead, many patients experience symptom relief through lifestyle and dietary changes and adopting alternative therapies. There are countless alternative therapies, too long to list in detail. The following are the most common therapies and lifestyle practices benefiting postcholecystectomy patients.

Chinese Medicine

It is thought that when bile does not flow properly, "liver qi stagnation" occurs. Qi (pronounced chē) is the circulating life force whose existence and properties are the basis of Chinese philosophy and medicine. The most popular Chinese medicine treatments involve points throughout the body known as meridians.

According to Asian medical philosophy, activation of these points with pressure (or needles) can improve blood flow, release tension, and enhance or unblock qi. This release allows energy to flow more freely through the meridians, promoting relaxation, healing and the restoration of proper function.

In Chinese medicine, the energetic functions of the gallbladder are:

Store and mobilize bile for digestion
Promote physical coordination and agility
Maintain health of connective tissues
Balances liver energy
Confer decision-making ability
Promote courage and initiative
Defensive energy against catching infections

Therefore, when the gallbladder is removed, a disruption in some or all of these functions may occur. To remedy this shift in the body's qi, several approaches may be employed by a Chinese medicine practitioner. These include:

Acupressure—applying pressure to the various meridian points.
Acupuncture—insertion of very thin needles into various meridian points.
Cupping—suction cups placed on the body that purportedly improve blood flow and rev up the body's healing process.
Electroacupuncture—same as acupuncture, but a slight electrical current is applied to the needles.
Five Element Theory and/or Yin and Yang Theory—elements of these ancient medical theories are used to determine treatment protocols for physical and emotional health.
Herbal therapy—next to dietary therapy, is perhaps the most widely used Traditional Chinese Medicine treatment modality. There are over 5,000 medicinal substances currently in use, including plant, animal, and mineral substances. Practitioners typically "prescribe" decoctions, which are specific herbal combinations for various ailments.
Moxibustion—dried plant materials called "moxa" are burned on or very near the surface of the skin to warm and invigorate the flow of qi in the body and dispel toxins.

Qigong—integrates physical postures, breathing techniques and focused intention.

Shiatsu—pressure with thumbs, hands, elbows, knees or feet is applied to pressure points on the body.

Tai Chi—involves a series of gentle exercise movements performed in a slow, focused manner and accompanied by deep breathing.

Tuina—a therapeutic, manipulative form of massage.

Essential Oils

I've met several postcholecystectomy patients who swear by essential oils for just about every ailment. They are easy to use, but be cautious as they are highly concentrated and strong. Finding a practitioner well-versed in essential oils is recommended. Essential oils seem innocent enough but due to their potency may cause adverse reactions in some people.

A drop or two of an essential oil is generally applied to the feet or belly area. You can also add a couple drops to a carrier oil like grapeseed oil, avocado oil, or my favorite combination—organic wheat germ and jojoba oil. I recommend buying organic essential and carrier oils where the herbs and soil were not sprayed with pesticides.

Go slow with essential oils and be cautious. There are many Internet resources available for researching which oils help with which ailments. Search for these essential oil qualities: antispasmodic, anti-nausea, anti-inflammatory and digestive.

Ayurveda

Ayurveda is a 5,000-year-old system of natural healing from India. It relies on multiple regimens to attain health and includes building a healthy metabolic system and maintaining good digestion and excretion, lifestyle, yoga, meditation, life-affirming mental attitude, therapies as well as Ayurvedic medicine. Ayurvedic professionals use the five senses to diagnose and some therapies rely on herbal compounds. To find an Ayurveda professional, you can search on the Internet or contact local holistic wellness and naturopathic centers.

Castor Oil Packs

The first naturopath I saw for my postcholecystectomy symptoms recommended I apply castor oil packs daily for my symptoms. It didn't help me all that much, but I figured I would put it in here as some people say it helped their digestive symptoms. The reported medicinal uses of castor oil packs are: drawing impurities from the liver, improving circulation, draining the lymphatic system, and combatting inflammation.

This is how I made my castor oil pack: 1. Cut a piece of flannel so it is big enough to cover your right upper quadrant (half of the front part of your abdomen and half of the back around the right ribs). 2. Drench the flannel in a high-grade non-toxic brand of castor oil. 3. Apply the flannel to the right upper quadrant and wrap saran plastic wrap around your torso and the flannel to hold it in place and keep it covered and protected. 4. Finally, apply a large heating pad to the entire area.

Regardless if it really works, it was a very relaxing treatment. Therefore, whether it truly can heal postcholecystectomy syndrome, at least you will be relaxed and your skin smoother. A word of caution is not to use castor oil packs if you are pregnant. Castor oil is reported to induce labor.

Biofeedback

This type of therapy is typically done with a mental health therapist but can be self-administered through computer programs. During a biofeedback session, electrodes are attached to your skin which record your heart and breathing rate, blood pressure, skin temperature, sweating, and/or muscle activity. When you are under stress or experience pain, it will show on the monitor. A biofeedback therapist, or the computer program, will help you practice relaxation exercises, which will be practiced coinciding with monitoring your different bodily functions with the goal of pain and stress relief, and improved wellbeing.

Reiki

Reiki is based on qi. It is a form of hands-on-healing. The reiki practitioner transfers their positive energy to the recipient which encourages healing. Reiki addresses physical, emotional, mental, and spiritual imbalances.

Until a few years ago, I thought reiki was ridiculously fake and hokey. In 2012, I had reiki performed on me by volunteers while I was a patient in the hospital. After, I felt no better or worse. A few years later, I had several reiki sessions and every time, at the end of the treatment, I'd feel a shift in my energy level and cried for no reason other than it was cleansing. As the day went on, my pain lessened.

Now, I believe in reiki. My local food co-op has reiki volunteers who donate their time, so it was free for me to sign up for a ½ hour session. Even if it was solely a placebo effect, I did feel better after each session.

Visceral massage

Visceral massage is a type of massage that targets the area between the skin, muscles, and internal organs, sometimes actually massaging the organ (externally of course). Some postcholecystectomy patients have had visceral massage sessions targeting the gallbladder and sphincter of Oddi area who say it helped improve their symptoms.

It is believed non-muscular organs like the kidneys, liver, stomach, intestines, pancreas, etc. can harden and inhibit blood flow. It is also thought organs can form trigger points, which are thought to be points of local tenderness to broader areas, referring pain and/or tension elsewhere. Visceral massage is often used to heal adhesions (scar tissue) deeply embedded around a surgical area that may have spread.

Bioidentical Hormones

It is estimated that 75 to 98% of patients suffering from SOD are women who had their gallbladders removed. This alone points to the likelihood hormones affect our liver and biliary system since such a large majority of sufferers are women. Often, women report a cessation of their SOD symptoms during pregnancy, only to have them reawaken post-partum.

Bioidentical hormones are not to be confused with prescription birth control or hormone replacement therapy. Bioidentical hormones are usually prescribed by a natural health practitioner and made at a compounding pharmacy. You can also acquire these creams pre-compounded at health food and drug stores, and on the Internet.

A practitioner will prescribe bioidentical hormones based on symptomology or a blood and/or saliva hormone test of progesterone, estrogen, DHEA, cortisol, and testosterone. I know a few women with postcholecystectomy pain who reported that after applying a compound of progesterone and estrogen or progesterone-alone, their symptoms eased. Progesterone is well-documented to relax the biliary sphincter and may control spasms. More information about hormones and their effect on the digestive system is described in Chapter 10.

Breathing, Meditation, and Yoga

Some may wonder how activities like meditation and breathing help postcholecystectomy syndrome. The fact is stress, anxiety, and depression impact our digestive system and pain perception. No, I am not insinuating your symptoms are all in your head. One of my biggest pet peeves is to learn of a patient's health care provider suggesting their symptoms are purely psychological. However, stress and emotional imbalance could make things worse and impede recovery or remission. Therefore, it is important to treat our minds along with the rest of our bodies.

I can't tell you how many times I felt sick, then became stressed over being sick, then felt sicker because I was stressed, then felt more stressed because I was feeling sicker. This went on and on. It was a vicious cycle. Rather than feed into fear and a negative stress response, get a handle on stress. It can help prevent symptoms from spiraling out of control.

Before my postcholecystectomy symptoms became disabling in 2011, I led a productive, healthy, low-pain life for 12 years following gallbladder surgery. Relying on deep breathing exercises, meditation, yoga, diet, and lifestyle changes kept my symptoms manageable. You may never be completely rid of pain or other symptoms, but these practices can help move them from the center stage of your life to the distant balcony.

One of the most valuable and easy remedies to practice is deep conscious breathing. In addition to sustaining our lives, amazing things happen on the cellular level when we breathe. Breathing deeply and with intention has shown to relieve stress and lessen pain. Though you breathe several times during each minute of the day when is the last time you paid attention to the way you breathe?

Think about the popular childbirth breathing program, Lamaze. According to the Lamaze International website, conscious breathing (especially slow breathing) reduces heart rate, anxiety, and pain perception. It works in part because when breathing becomes a focus, other sensations, such as labor pain, move to the edge of your awareness. Conscious breathing also keeps the expectant mom and baby "well oxygenated."

Recently, I came across a great article in Yoga Journal called, "The Science of Breathing." Fast, uneven breathing triggers the nervous system, turning up stress hormones, heart rate, blood pressure, muscle tension, sweat production, and anxiety. Alternatively, slowing your breath dials down all the above as it turns up relaxation, calm, and mental clarity. The deep inhales of conscious breathing introduce more oxygen into your body while deep release exhales remove the carbon dioxide waste products. In theory, more blood can be oxygenated using this technique.

So how does this help postcholecystectomy patients? Aside from what I just wrote, I don't know. I *do* know that once I began practicing conscious breathing, my postcholecystectomy pain became manageable. The pain did not disappear. It became tolerable. Through my breathing practice, I could achieve a level of acceptance and patience around my painful condition. Prior to this, I was living in fight or flight mode, making the pain worse. Today, I continue to practice this type of breathing especially when stressed, worried or scared.

Conscious breathing is simple. My only suggestion is to breathe deeply through your nose rather than your mouth. You will know you are doing it right when you make a slight hissing type sound, sort of like a light snore, at the base of your sinuses and be-ginning of your throat. Perform deep inhales for a count of at least four. You will want to fill your upper belly on inhale and deflate it on exhale. When inhaling, your goal is to stretch out your diaphragm, which serves as the main muscle of respiration and is attached to the lower ribs. Follow with an identical count exhale.

Meditation is another great way to control pain and symptoms. For the longest time, I considered myself a meditation flunky. In vain, I accumulated a rather large collection of books on meditation, including, "Meditation for Dummies," and viewed countless tutorials on how to meditate. Meditation alluded me for a very long time. Sitting still and quieting my mind was a constant struggle. Instead of clearing my head I would obsess over needing to vacuum the floor I was sitting on, or wonder if I set the DVR to record my favorite show. I would also get uncomfortable sitting straight up. I'd slouch and readjust my leg fold to get comfortable, but to no avail.

Finally, I realized I was never going to be perfect at meditation, and that was ok. I accepted the fact meditation was a lifelong work in progress. I changed my seated position to whatever position I felt comfortable, even if that meant lying down or curled up on the couch. I recognized the disruptive thoughts and imagined ushering them out of my mind without judgment. "Goodbye thought," I'd say to myself. I incorporated humming, chanting, my deep breathing practice. I still do not meditate perfectly or as often as would benefit me, but I'm doing my best, and that's what matters.

Most days I take advantage of guided meditations to lead me to a place of peace. You can order guided meditations online. I prefer to search for free guided meditations on YouTube and listen to the videos. I also have a few meditation apps downloaded onto my phone. Some people prefer podcasts.

To accelerate my meditation practice, I attended group meditation gatherings at our city's local Buddhist center. They were an hour long and led by an experienced group meditation leader. The leader read something then we meditated in a chair or on the floor for a half hour, followed by a slow walking meditation, and ending with a sitting meditation and a final reading. I started going because I knew if I went then I'd have to sit there and meditate. Sure enough, my theory worked.

A few years ago, I saw a certified hypnotist/hypnotherapist to strengthen my meditation practice and help me cope with my chronic pancreatitis pain. It was very helpful. I still use some of the self-talk the therapist taught me to relax and focus on absolutely nothing.

Another form of meditation is mindfulness meditation, which can be used while eating a meal. I have a friend who eats very slowly. Instead of getting annoyed over how long it would take her to finish her lunch or dinner while dining at a restaurant, I admired the way she ate with such intention and care. She would savor every morsel of food as I inhaled a whole plate of food within minutes. I have always been a fast eater, someone who ate like it was their last meal. My dad would say I ate, "like it was going out of style."

I realized that overeating and stuffing my face made my symptoms worse. It put an incredible strain on organs already strained from not having a gallbladder. I saw a naturopath who suggested I change the way I ate. She called it, "food hygiene," and told me to chew my food 20 or more times and count as I chewed. I did this for a few weeks, then reverted to my animalistic flare for eating.

To control my fast eating style, I began reading up on mindfulness meditation for eating. I thought mindfulness and meditation were one and the same, but they are different. With mindfulness, you focus and set your intention on one thing. For example, this could be breathing, an object, imagined a ball of color, or even a soothing word. This will lead you to a state of meditation in most instances.

As in meditation, you get comfortable and acknowledge disruptive thoughts, then shoo them away. But with mindfulness, you are aware of your intention. Your senses are highly alert. With breathing you would focus in on the air entering your nose and lungs, the smell of the air, the feeling of your lungs filling and diaphragm stretching. You become in tune with whatever it is you are focusing on. You could replicate this exercise with, for example, the sun—sitting in the sun and feeling its warmth and brightness through your eyes. With words, you can say a soothing word repeatedly, like serenity, calm, or peace. Mindfulness is the ultimate practice for being present in the moment.

There are several books and websites dedicated to teaching you how to practice mindful eating. With mindful eating, you set your intention on the food you are about to eat. Take a piece of fruit. Hold it in your hand. Say a prayer of thanks for the food you are about to consume. Then hold the food to your nose and release your sense of smell. Eat the food slowly, moving it around your mouth. Notice the texture and taste. Chew slowly then swallow.

Make eating a process, rather than a shovel fest. You can incorporate counting your chews if you want. If your focus is on the slow process of acknowledging and engaging the food you eat. Many dietitians are touting mindfulness eating as a weight loss strategy. This may concern some of you who have unintentionally lost weight due to your symptoms. I doubt you would lose much weight with mindfulness eating unless you also changed the food you were eating. Therefore, practicing it shouldn't detrimentally affect your weight.

In addition to breathing and meditation, I found yoga to be incredibly helpful. Yoga is a Hindu spiritual discipline, a part of which, including breath control, simple meditation, and the adoption of specific bodily postures, is widely practiced for health and relaxation. There are even specific poses to regenerate and relax the digestive system.

If it's your first time trying yoga, I strongly recommend attending a beginner's class before embarking on your own. Receiving proper yoga instruction ensures you are performing the poses correctly, which can prevent injury. You want to be sure you are benefiting from the poses, not making matters worse. The yoga instructor may also know of digestive-specific poses that could help alleviate your symptoms.

Yoga is offered in yoga studios, churches, community centers, gyms, and many other places. I even did something called Hiking Yoga in New York City's Central Park. Keep trying different classes until you find one you like. Also, find a yoga teacher that meets your individual needs. I definitely prefer some yoga teachers over others.

Once you have learned the basics of yoga, you can practice at home from memory or with a visual instructional aid. I own several yoga DVDs and still watch a pregnancy yoga video I practiced during my third pregnancy. I just happen to like the yoga teacher's calming demeanor and choice of poses. I also own one specifically meant for people with digestive issues. I generally steer clear of hardcore yoga DVDs meant for weight loss. It kind of defeats the purpose of yoga for stress relief if the yoga teacher is yelling at me to "feel the burn."

You can find a plethora of free yoga tutorials on YouTube and the Internet. Search using terms like, "yoga for the digestive system", "yoga poses for the liver or pancreas", or "relaxing yoga". There is no shortage of information on yoga poses for digestion. Yoga is a wonderful tool for grounding, relaxation, meditating, deep breathing and strengthening the muscles surrounding our digestive system.

Physical Exercise

Physical exercise is not only beneficial for your body's overall well-being, studies show it is especially good for your liver. Specifically, physical exercise reduces the risk of scarring and cirrhosis, fatty liver disease, muscle atrophy from significant weight loss; and improves blood sugar and insulin levels, depression and anxiety, blood oxygenation, and energy.

For some postcholecystectomy patients, however, physical exercise triggers their symptoms. I have had this personally happen to me numerous times when I engaged in high interval training exercises. A few people I met in the support groups complained of the same thing. Every time they ran or did aerobics, they would experience a symptom flare-up.

Therefore, please do not perform an exercise that will cause or intensify pain or other symptoms. It isn't worth it. I know it is difficult to give up something you love, but it is also traumatic to deal with severe pain and puts unhealthy stress on the body and mind. It is well known that pain increases blood pressure and can even cause shock.

Find a healthy activity with the benefits of cardiovascular and muscle toning that doesn't leave you screaming in pain. Work on finding exercises that help your symptoms and only then should you reintroduce high impact exercises gradually.

There are many varieties of activities you could try that don't necessarily involve a gym membership. For example, I enjoy walking outside, kayaking and hiking. My parents were avid hikers, so I grew up hiking mountains and trails. I bought a quality pair of hiking boots so I wouldn't be in pain from sore feet. Quality footwear for any exercise or physical activity is important and worth the investment.

Cycling may be a good activity. I just wouldn't recommend an intense spinning class if you want to avoid flare-ups. Swimming is another great way to get a full body workout without putting too much stress on your body. Whatever you do, get off that couch and do something! Of course, if you were as sick as me during my worst year, I was too weak to do much of anything and couldn't afford to lose weight from exercising. If this is the case, stick with very gentle stretching, yoga or Tai Chi.

Chapter 6: Medications

Medications can be beneficial for alleviating a variety of postcholecystectomy symptoms and conditions. The first course of treatment a physician commonly takes for postcholecystectomy symptoms, after diet and lifestyle modifications fail, is prescribing a medication. Ideally, doctors would exhaust all medication options before advancing to an invasive treatment option.

As I described in Chapter 2, there are numerous conditions related to postcholecystectomy syndrome. Rather than list treatments for each condition, I will focus on describing the most common medications used for the most common postcholecystectomy symptoms and conditions.

These medications are listed by their United States generic drug names. If you are from a different country, you should easily be able to find their counterparts by searching online. This is by no means a complete list. It is likely with new drugs always on the horizon and others not available in the U.S. or in other countries, I may have unintentionally omitted effective drugs.

Bile Acid Sequestrants

Bile acid sequestrants are commonly prescribed for bile acid diarrhea and bile acid malabsorption. These medications bind to bile acids, forming a non-absorbable complex. This reduces damage to the intestinal mucosa, induction of colonic fluid secretion, which causes watery diarrhea and inhibits reabsorption of intestinal bile salts. Since there is a reduction in bile that is reabsorbed, the liver will make new bile.

These medications can also help patients suffering from bile reflux as the sequestrant begins to bind with bile present in the stomach, sweeping it out of the stomach.

Doctors also use bile acid sequestrants to lower their patients' bad cholesterol levels. Since bile acids are synthesized from cholesterol, disruption of bile acid reabsorption will decrease cholesterol levels, particularly the amount of LDL cholesterol (bad cholesterol) circulating in the blood. Therefore, if you have very low cholesterol levels, you may not be able to take this medication.

Examples of bile acid sequestrants are:

Cholestyramine (comes in a powder form to be mixed in water or juice)
Colesevelam (comes in pill form)
Colestipol (comes in pill form)

Since bile acid sequestrants are designed to stay in the gut, they generally do not have systemic side effects. However, they may cause problems in the gastrointestinal tract, such as constipation and flatulence.

Bile acid sequestrants may also bind with other medications and vitamins, preventing their absorption into the bloodstream. Therefore, it is generally advised that bile acid sequestrants be spaced several hours apart from other drugs and supplements. Most concerning is these medications may bind fat-soluble vitamins, such as vitamins A, D, E, and K. This effect may result in a vitamin deficiency and supplementation may be warranted.

Ursodeoxycholic acid

Ursodeoxycholic acid is a chemical naturally occurring in bile and can be used to dissolve gallstones. This medication blocks the enzyme in the liver that produces cholesterol and thereby decreases the production of cholesterol by the liver and the amount of cholesterol in bile. This medication may be used to dissolve microscopic gallstones and "thin" the bile. It is the only drug that is FDA-approved to treat primary biliary cirrhosis.

Postcholecystectomy patients experiencing thick sludge-like bile may benefit from taking ursodeoxycholic acid. Caution should always be taken as this medication can cause a blockage when thinned-out bile encounters gallstones or sludge.

Prescription Pancreatic Enzymes (pancrealipase)

In the previous chapter, I explained the benefit of taking over the counter digestive enzymes and defined amylase, protease, and lipase—the ingredients in prescription pancreatic enzymes. Various strengths and brands are available, but all prescription enzymes are made from pigs, which could be a problem for vegans or vegetarians.

When my postcholecystectomy symptoms became horribly problematic after the birth of my third son, I developed a whole cadre of new symptoms. One that was horribly painful originated from my pancreas. I didn't think anything could be worse than the postcholecystectomy pain I had for years in my right side. Then I was introduced to pancreatic pain, a constant searing pain under my sternum that sometimes radiated to my left side and back.

I suffered without treatment for six months before a gastroenterologist finally thought a prescription of enzymes could help. A week after taking my first pill, the pain was nearly gone. I still take them and still have pancreatic pain, but the enzymes help to absorb food, which gives my pancreas a break.

Not everyone with postcholecystectomy syndrome needs prescription-strength enzymes. These medications should be reserved for patients with pancreatic gallstones, chronic pancreatitis, pancreatic sphincter disorder, exocrine pancreatic deficiency, or other pancreatic conditions. If you experience excessive bloating and gas while taking enzymes, you may need a smaller dose or a different brand.

Anticholinergics and Antispasmodics

Anticholinergics interfere with the action of the neurochemical acetylcholine and block involuntary movements. They stop the transmission of parasympathetic nerve impulses, therefore, lessening the spasms of smooth muscle, such as in the gastrointestinal tract and in the bladder. Most antispasmodic agents are also anticholinergics. They can work directly on the smooth muscle in the wall of the gut. Here they help to relax the muscle and relieve the pain associated with a contraction of the gut.

Since the sphincter of Oddi is a tiny smooth muscle, it is thought this class of drugs will prevent the sphincter from spasm and quell the nerve pain associated with SOD. It may also help alleviate biliary spasm, IBS symptoms, and nerve pain. I have witnessed many postcholecystectomy patients gain relief by taking this class of drugs. Side effects are generally minimal, but for some become intolerable. The most common are mucous membrane dryness, dizziness, and drowsiness.

Examples of anticholinergic or antispasmodic agents are hyoscyamine, chlordiazepoxide (clidinium), dicyclomine, scopolamine, glycopyrrolate, amitriptyline, nortriptyline, atropine, mebeverine (not available in the U.S.), and combinations of these generics with phenobarbital and belladonna.

Muscle Relaxants

Muscle relaxants are agents that reduce tension in muscles. Centrally acting muscle relaxants work by reducing the tone of skeletal muscle causing muscles to relax. These are generally used to relieve skeletal muscle spasms due to spastic conditions, and can be used to relieve musculoskeletal pain. Some muscle relaxants also work by blocking pain sensations between the nerves and the brain.

Like the anticholinergic/antispasmodic class of drugs, muscle relaxants are prescribed to stop the sphincter of Oddi, bile duct and/or bowel from spasm. Examples of muscle relaxants are cyclobenzaprine, carisoprodol, baclofen, and buscopan. Common side effects are similar to anticholinergics and antispasmodics.

Calcium Channel Blockers

Calcium channel blockers are typically used to treat high blood pressure and heart conditions. They act as a smooth muscle selective calcium channel antagonists and potent inhibitors of sphincter of Oddi contractions. This medication is particularly helpful when a patient is having a painful SOD attack, which is typically a stabbing pain under the right ribcage. Regardless if you have SOD or not, this drug could help quell postcholecystectomy pain in the upper right quadrant.

The downside is its effect on blood pressure. If someone has low or even normal blood pressure, these medications can cause a severe drop in blood pressure. If you do not have low blood pressure and experience sudden pain attacks, you may want to discuss this medication with your doctor.

Examples of calcium channel blockers are nitroglycerin, nifedipine, diltiazem, amlodipine, and felodipine.

Anti-epileptic Anticonvulsant Medications

This class of drugs was created to mimic some of the effects of GABA, an inhibitory neurotransmitter found in the central nervous system (CNS) that regulates its excitability. These drugs are used with other medications to prevent and control seizures. They are also used to relieve nerve pain. Some gastroenterologists believe postcholecystectomy pain is a neuralgia, which is pain from damaged nerves.

Prescribing of these drugs for pain conditions has become popular in the pain management community. In addition to relieving nerve pain, they are often used as an alternative to narcotic pain medications like opioids. Drugs in this class are gabapentin and forms of gabapentin, i.e. pregabalin and gabapentin enacarbil. These drugs can make you very drowsy or groggy.

Anti-nausea (Antiemetic) Medications

Anti-nausea/Antiemetic medications are used to control nausea and vomiting. If nausea and vomiting are uncontrollable, oral therapy may not be appropriate and intravenous administration at a hospital may be necessary. Alternatively, some of these medications are available in suppository form for home use.

The first type of anti-nausea/antiemetic medication is the 5-HT3 receptor antagonist, which blocks serotonin receptors in the central nervous system and gastrointestinal tract. The most common 5-HT3 receptor antagonist prescribed for nausea is ondansetron. This drug was once reserved for cancer patients receiving chemotherapy but is now widely used for any type of nausea syndrome, including morning sickness during pregnancy. It is most useful because it is non-sedating.

Mirtazapine is another example of a 5-HT3 receptor antagonist. However, it is quite sedating and primarily prescribed as an anti-depressant.

The second type of anti-nausea/antiemetic agents is dopamine antagonists. These block the body's dopamine receptors. The most commonly prescribed in this class are metoclopramide and domperidone. These are also "pro-kinetics", which increase gut motility and can help alleviate symptoms of gastroparesis (slow gut motility).

It baffles me that domperidone is not FDA-approved in the U.S., but metoclopramide is. Some of metoclopramide's side effects are serious and dangerous, including tardive dyskinesia, irregular blood pressure, and neuroleptic disorders. However, I have met a few patients who take metoclopramide with no side effects. Simply use caution with this medication and alert your doctor of any strange effects.

Apparently, domperidone was not been approved in the U.S. because it caused heart irregularities in those receiving it intravenously in very large amounts. It also raises levels of the hormone prolactin, which is why some breastfeeding moms use it to increase their milk supply. Prolactin triggers milk production, but high prolactin levels have been linked to pituitary gland tumors. When I was taking it regularly, I had my prolactin levels monitored by my doctor.

In the U.S., domperidone can be acquired by prescription, but must be filled at a compounding pharmacy. There are also several websites where it can be ordered overseas. In most countries, domperidone can be purchased over the counter. My domperidone was prescribed by a local gastroenterologist. However, it was too costly to purchase through a compounding pharmacy. All I will say is I got my domperidone one way or another and thanked God every day I had it on hand when I needed it for nausea and to relieve the "full feeling" in my gut. The only side effect I experienced was a slight increase in my foot neuropathy, but it was worth the nausea relief.

Other medications used to control nausea are H1 histamine receptor antagonists (antihistamines). Unfortunately, these medications cause drowsiness. Over the counter brands are diphenhydramine, meclizine, and dimenhydrinate. The more sedating brands require a prescription, ex. promethazine and hydroxyzine.

Irritable Bowel Syndrome (IBS) Medications

Before I describe the most common IBS medications, it is important I warn you to *never*, I repeat, *never*, take eluxadoline (brand name is Viberzi) if you had your gallbladder removed. In the U.S., the FDA has issued a warning regarding this product. It is contraindicated in patients with no gallbladder and those with pancreatitis. Several deaths have occurred as the result of postcholecystectomy patients taking this drug. Most of these deaths resulted from the drug causing acute pancreatitis.

IBS is usually a diagnosis of exclusion in patients with unexplained bowel symptoms like diarrhea, constipation, and/or intestinal pain. Once intestinal conditions such as bile acid diarrhea, Crohn's disease, diverticulitis, celiac disease, infection, SIBO, or obstruction have been ruled out, your doctor may diagnose you with IBS.

Those who suffer from IBS-D (IBS with diarrhea) generally experience frequent loose or watery stools with abdominal pain. The abdominal pain is associated with a change in the frequency or consistency of stool. The altered bowel habit may be as frequent as several times a day or only occur once a day. Bloating or distention in the abdomen is also common.

The most popular IBS-D medications are anti-diarrheals, including atropine, diphenoxylate, and loperamide which may be acquired by prescription or over-the-counter. These should be reserved for severe instances of diarrhea and used for a limited time as some studies reported patients developing a physical dependence on them. Therefore, when the patient ceases treatment, their symptoms return and, in some cases, worsen.

Alosetron, a 5-HT3 antagonist, is FDA-approved for IBS-D. It may relieve abdominal pain and slow colonic and small bowel transit. Alosetron was withdrawn from the market for safety reasons in 2000, including ischemic colitis and complications of constipation, and was reintroduced in 2002 with greater restrictions. Specific guidelines for the use of alosetron require doctors who prescribe it to sign a certificate and patients to sign a consent form.

Rifaximin is an antibiotic that was FDA-approved for the treatment of IBS-D. Altering the colonic bacterial flora and reducing bad bacteria with this medication has reduced IBS-D symptoms in some patients. This drug is also used to treat SIBO with or without constipation or diarrhea. Rifaximin has been shown to help people who have diarrhea and bloating as their worst symptoms. Rifaximin can be taken for 14 days. People who have symptoms again can be retreated for 14 days. This can be done one more time if needed.

Budesonide is a glucocorticoid steroid medication that stays in your intestines rather than affect your entire body like other steroids. It works as an anti-inflammatory by decreasing the body's natural immune response. It can be useful to control diarrhea associated with IBS, inflammatory bowel syndromes, and microscopic colitis. Due to limited systemic availability, steroidal side effects are minimal.

IBS-C (IBS with constipation) is another form of IBS. Patients generally experience abdominal pain, bloating or discomfort associated with constipation. Stools are hard or lumpy, and the patient may go days without having a bowel movement. IBS-C medications primarily focus on loosening stools or increasing their water content. Take them with care as you can develop the opposite problem—diarrhea—if your dose is incorrect.

Osmotic laxatives increase the water content in the intestine to assist with fecal elimination. Milk of Magnesia is an osmotic laxative that absorbs water from the blood to the intestine. It increases the water content of the undigested food and provides a flushing action on the stool. Another osmotic laxative is lactulose, a synthetic sugar syrup you must obtain by prescription. It breaks down in your large intestine and draws water into the intestine. This softens your stool, which helps ease constipation.

Stimulant laxatives (such as senokot or bisacodyl) induce a bowel movement by acting to speed up colonic muscle movement (motility). Your body can become dependent on stimulant laxatives. Therefore, they should only be used temporarily.

Stool softeners (such as docusate sodium and docusate calcium) increase the water capacity of stools. The softened stool allows the body to evacuate it more easily than hardened stool.

Linaclotide is a prescription medication that is a guanylate cyclase-C agonist. It works by increasing the amount of fluid in the intestines, causing the contents to evacuate more quickly.

Lubiprostone is a prescription medication belonging to a class of drugs known as chloride channel activators. It works by increasing the amount of fluid within your intestines, making the passage of stool easier.

Medical Marijuana

Medical marijuana is becoming a popular treatment for pain, nausea, and many other ailments. I know quite a few postcholecystectomy patients who say they wouldn't be able to work or function if not for medical marijuana or marijuana derivatives. They laud its miraculous ability to improve pain, nausea, anxiety, stress, etc.

Of course, one major problem with medical marijuana is that it isn't legal everywhere so the pot you just purchased from your brother in law's "connection" may not be an appropriate strain for your symptoms. Also, the stuff you get off the street was likely sprayed with lots of chemicals, which you will be inhaling or ingesting, whereas medical marijuana is organically grown or grown using few chemical additives.

If you purchase medical marijuana under the guidance of your physician, your chance of obtaining a "perfect match" strain for your symptoms increases dramatically. I wouldn't attempt to recommend a strain and will leave that up to the experts.

You may, however, consider a low THC strain if you want to function fully during the day and leave the higher THC marijuana strains for evening use. THC is the ingredient owing to the marijuana "high". CBD is another substance in marijuana which aids nausea and pain. But, CBD alone will not benefit all symptoms. You can, though, acquire a balanced CBD/THC strain or a high CBD/low THC strain.

If you use marijuana medicinally, be careful ingesting it as it could exacerbate your digestive issues. Vaporizing or using an oil or tincture may be the best option.

Opioid Pain Medication

Most opioid pain medications carry "spasm of sphincter of Oddi" as a side effect. They are also notorious for causing constipation and slowing gut motility. Opioid pain medication is meant for acute pain and short-term use. However, anyone who has had a severe chronic pain condition knows that may not be realistic and opioid treatment difficult to obtain.

There are several dilemmas these drugs present, including their addictive nature (and subsequent withdrawal syndrome), the opiophobic trend of doctors, and criminalization of these drugs. Many pain management and primary care doctors will not prescribe opioid pain medication under any circumstances, which often leaves it to hospital emergency rooms to act as pain management programs. Instead, the growing trend has been for pain doctors to push steroid injections and spinal cord stimulators.

If you are prescribed opioid pain medication, take as minimal a dose as possible, but work with your doctor on determining what that is. I have seen too many patients build up a tolerance to pain medication to the point their doctors don't feel comfortable prescribing the amount they are on. Also, when tolerance is too high, and you go into a flare, intravenous doses of pain medication administered in the hospital may not get the pain under control.

Opioids also produce hyperalgesia—an increased sensitivity to pain. In other words, pain meds can cause more pain over time.

Naloxone/Low Dose Naltrexone

Naloxone, an opiate blocker used to treat opioid overdoses and as an opioid withdrawal aid, has been shown to reverse opioid-induced sphincter of Oddi spasms and relieve pain conditions. There are, though, only a few case studies about this and those studies were based on opioid-dependent patients. It certainly is a drug worthy of future studies.

Low-dose naltrexone (LDN) has a similar chemical composition to naloxone, but is generally longer-acting. It acts as an immune-modulator and is emerging as a treatment for IBS and autoimmune conditions like Crohn's disease, celiac, ulcerative colitis, and primary biliary cirrhosis. In the U.S., LDN must be obtained by prescription and filled at a compounding pharmacy. You may have trouble finding a physician who will prescribe LDN as it is a fairly new treatment.

I developed microscopic colitis, probably from bile malabsorption or overuse of NSAID medications like ibuprofen. LDN took care of the associated symptoms when no other medication worked. Though there are few side effects, over time I developed abdominal cramps from this drug. However, for the six months I took it, my symptoms, primarily diarrhea, and weight loss, were relieved.

Benzodiazepines

According to the National Library of Medicine, benzodiazepines are a large class of medications that have multiple clinical uses including therapy of anxiety, insomnia, muscle spasm, alcohol withdrawal, and seizures. The pharmacological effects of the benzodiazepines are a result of their interaction with the central nervous system, their effects being sedation, hypnosis, decreased anxiety, muscle relaxation, anterograde amnesia and anticonvulsant activity.

Benzodiazepines can be very useful drugs for nausea, vomiting, dizziness, some digestive ailments, and to ameliorate the stress and anxiety associated with chronic illness. Sounds like a wonder drug, right? Let me tell you, they are not. The downside is benzodiazepines are highly addictive. Meaning, they are a bitch to come off if you've been on them a while. And, your tolerance levels of the drug can build up, so you require more and more. The horror stories of interdose withdrawal and withdrawal syndrome are prevalent on the Internet. These drugs are best used for short periods or on occasion. In fact, it is widely documented that these medications are not recommended beyond a few weeks.

If it weren't for the temporary use of benzodiazepines when my symptoms disabled me, I would have lost my mind. The most useful aspect was its effect on my nausea and vomiting. Unfortunately, like with most benzos, my body became dependent. It was hell coming off them and in the end, I believe this class of drugs was to blame for inducing pancreatitis episodes. I tested this theory by going on and off them, each time my pancreatitis got worse.

Coming off medications can produce side effects just as bad or worse than the actual drug can. I have met several people who experienced severe digestive symptoms while tapering off this medication or were experiencing interdose withdrawal. Some experienced protracted withdrawal symptoms months and years after stopping the drug. Many people I know on benzodiazepines have mystery digestive ailments. Since these drugs bind to GABA receptors, which are prevalent throughout the digestive tract and organs, digestion will naturally be affected either positively or negatively by these medications or from their withdrawal. Use caution when taking them and consider reserving them for occasional use and not long-term.

Birth Control Pills

There are quite a few women who claim their postcholecystectomy digestive symptoms and pain went away when they are on birth control and cannot go off it without having severe symptoms return. There are also women who developed digestive symptoms by going on birth control or hormone replacement therapy.

There is very little consistency or predictability when it comes to hormone therapy and its effects on postcholecystectomy symptoms. Birth control that seems to be the most effective for helping postcholecystectomy symptoms is one that is a low dose of both estrogen and progesterone or progesterone alone. Some women who have been diagnosed "estrogen dominant" claim remission of their postcholecystectomy symptoms after taking a progesterone-only pill or using progesterone cream. More about hormones is described in Chapter 10.

Medication Safety and Side Effects

I was the type of person who relied on pills to cure whatever ailed me. Had a headache? Took a pill. Felt sad? Went to the doctor to get a pill. Had a slight infection? Hurry up and get an antibiotic. Now I run far away from a prescription pad unless I know a medicine will save my life or greatly improve my quality of life, and not disable or kill me in the process.

This change in attitude came at a price after I had a severe long term adverse reaction to a fluoroquinolone antibiotic, i.e., Cipro, Avelox, Levaquin. This reaction left me with severe neuropathy, connective tissue problems, and a completely messed up central nervous system. And don't get me started on how sick I was coming off a benzodiazepine.

As of this writing, it has been four and a half years since I was given the fluoroquinolone antibiotic and some of my symptoms appear to be permanent. I never thought an antibiotic could do so much damage, but it did. Now there are black box warnings from the FDA about these drugs, not that I would have paid attention. I never thought severe side effects would happen to me. All those terrible potential side effects listed on the drug commercials happened to other people.

Keep in mind, most medications are metabolized in the liver where this organ's enzymes and detoxification pathways are responsible for converting medication to its active component and removing its associated toxins from the body. Ideally, this process runs smoothly with few problems. This, however, may not be the case for people without a gallbladder and a strained liver.

Additionally, genetic mutations can play a major role in how you tolerate a medication. I found an incredible amount of information relative to my genetics by consulting a natural health practitioner specializing in epigenetics/genomics. At her suggestion, I ordered DNA testing through www.23andme.com. After I received the results, she went over my genetic mutations and recommended a supplement, diet, and lifestyle plan for my genetic body type. She also explained why I struggled with certain medications in relation to my specific mutations.

My reason for mentioning all of this isn't to scare you completely away from medications, but to encourage you to be cautious with any prescription or over the counter medication you consider taking for your symptoms. Ask your doctor if there are black box warnings for a medication and what the most common side effects are for any drug. Get to know your pharmacist and let him or her know you want to be alerted of possible drug interactions and severe side effects.

Also, ask your pharmacist to alert you if a medication is contraindicated for people lacking a gallbladder. You may want to steer clear of drugs causing spasm of sphincter of Oddi or acute pancreatitis too. Remember, doctors and pharmacists don't always know every side effect, and many aren't listed in the product's post marketing materials.

I can't tell you how many times a doctor or pharmacist told me a strange symptom I was experiencing could not be from the drug I was taking. Consequently, I would cease taking the drug and the side effect would go away or improve. Therefore, always go with your gut instinct. There is a reason .0001% of people get a side effect, and the rest of the population don't. Everyone is unique and thanks to our genetics and liver enzymes we metabolize drugs differently.

Chapter 7: Procedural and Surgical Treatments

When all else fails, and postcholecystectomy symptoms are not improved with diet, medications or natural healing methods, more invasive measures may need to be considered. Going the procedural or surgical route is not a decision to be taken lightly. I have witnessed quite a few patients, including myself, come close to dying from acute pancreatitis, excessive bleeding, infections and other complications of procedures and surgeries.

Regardless, in some cases, procedures or surgeries are the only option for postcholecystectomy patients to have a quality and seemingly normal life. Arriving at the decision to have an invasive procedure or surgery is one that is usually born out of desperation. You would do just about anything to feel better, including risk your life. Some postcholecystectomy patients have such severe symptoms it is impossible for them to live a normal life. This could cause anyone to make a drastic, potentially life-changing decision, with the hope of getting better.

Just as I have witnessed the ill effects of invasive treatments, I have witnessed many success stories. Therefore, it is impossible to know who will benefit from which procedure. My surgery, a transduodenal sphincteroplasty, has afforded me a life nearly void of nausea and right-side pain. If I had to do it all over again, I would have surgery, though it was painful; and I developed a septic infection.

Please consider the following when deciding on a procedure or surgery:

What are the statistical chances this procedure/surgery will work for my symptoms and condition?
What risks are associated with the procedure/surgery, i.e. infection, bleeding, morbidity?
Do the risks outweigh the possible benefits?
How long will it take to recover from the procedure/surgery?
How will my pain be managed after the procedure/surgery?

If you are considering having an invasive procedure, I strongly suggest you join an online support group or forum associated with your condition to find out how others faired with that same procedure. Each person is different, but it may help you to make an informed decision. It will also give you a snapshot of best and worst-case scenarios.

It may frighten you to hear a story of a near death experience with a procedure you already have scheduled. But, it may force you to reconsider whether you really need the procedure and learn about precautions to consider if you go through with the procedure.

If you are determined to have an invasive procedure, you can also learn from others about what is a realistic recovery period. Doctors will give you an estimate of the number of days you will be hospitalized. If it is an outpatient procedure, find out the likelihood it could turn into an inpatient stay at the hospital. Though the doctor will have a good idea of how the procedure will go, fellow patients are still the best resource to gauge a realistic post-op recovery timeframe.

The following is a list of the most common procedures and surgeries performed for treating postcholecystectomy conditions.

Surgical Correction of Cholecystectomy Complications

Gallbladder surgery is never foolproof. Bile leak, injury to the bile duct, and slip of the surgical clips can occur. Symptoms related to this can appear immediately following surgery, several months, or years later. Most surgery-related complications can be diagnosed through scans or non-invasive procedures.

Injury to the bile duct and other organs can occur during surgery by the instruments or human error. Even the most talented surgeons can make mistakes. If this happens, further surgery may be needed.

When the gallbladder is removed, special clips are used to seal the tube that connects the gallbladder to the main bile duct. Normally, after the removal of the gallbladder, the remaining portion of the bile duct (the cystic duct) is clipped to prevent bile leaks and other complications. However, this clip may dislocate slightly, leading to pain and increased risk of bile leak in the abdominal area. In addition, rarely, patients are sensitive to the metal of the clip, which can be problematic.

A bile leak can be detected through an ERCP to follow the movement of bile. Repair procedures may be possible via a cut into the common bile duct and insertion of stents and/or a T-tube inserted during this procedure. The T-tube is shaped like the letter "T". This T-tube is inserted into the common bile duct while the bottom part drains out of the abdomen into a drainage bag. Stents will be described in the next section.

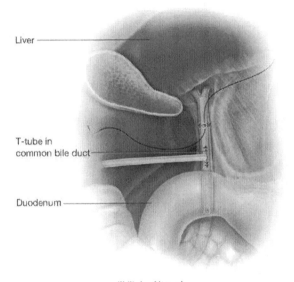

T Tube Visual

Stent Placement

Stents are placed into the bile or pancreatic duct to bypass strictures, or narrowed parts of the duct, allowing bile to flow better and help keep the sphincters wide and open. They may also help prevent biliary spasms/dyskinesia.

There are two types of stents that are commonly used. The first is made of plastic and looks like a small straw. The second type of stent is made of metal wires that look like the cross wires of a fence or cage. The metal stent is flexible, expandable and springs open to a larger diameter than plastic stents. Stents stent can be pushed through an ERCP scope into a blocked duct to allow normal drainage.

Both plastic and metal stents tend to clog up after several months and may require another ERCP to swap out the old stent for a new one. Metal stents are more permanent while plastic stents are easily removed at a repeat procedure. Your doctor will choose the best type of stent for your problem.

Pancreatic stents can help with SOD and pancreatic symptoms. However, their insertion may disturb the pancreas, which is temperamental and prone to inflammation. Stents are not ever meant to be permanent. And, though it may be a bother to get them routinely swapped out, it could be worth the hassle to avoid the risks of other, more invasive solutions. The risks of stent placement include acute pancreatitis (from pancreatic stent placement), ductal perforation, and any risks involved with anesthesia and endoscopy.

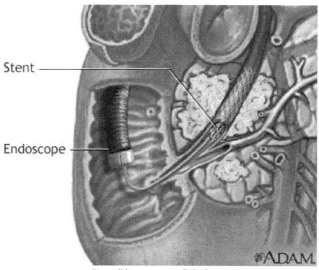

Stent Placement in Bile Duct

Balloon Dilatation/Dilation

Balloon dilatation is generally used to retrieve stones and sludge in the bile duct, but may also be performed for biliary strictures. During an ERCP, a physician will use a catheter fitted with a dilating balloon to stretch the sphincter and duct area. This balloon is inflated with a sterile saline solution up to a size (at least > 10 mm in diameter) and duration (usually 2–6 minutes) according to the patients' condition and tolerance. The balloon is then inflated to stretch out the narrowing. To minimize the risk of perforation, the size of the balloon should not exceed the size of the common bile duct.

Dilatation with balloons is often performed when the cause of the narrowing is benign (not cancerous). After balloon dilatation, a temporary stent may be placed for a few months to help maintain the dilation. Risks are the same for balloon dilatation as they are for stents. Also, the balloon could break and get stuck in the duct, which will, of course, need retrieval.

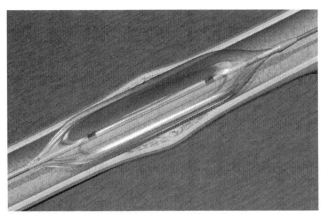

Balloon Dilatation in Biliary Duct

Sphincterotomy

Sphincterotomy is cutting of the biliary and pancreatic sphincter muscle. It is performed to open the sphincters in patients with SOD or strictures and to remove adhesions around the sphincter area. It is generally an outpatient procedure in which you will prepare as you would for an endoscopy and be sedated. The cut is made to enlarge

116

the opening while your doctor looks through an ERCP scope at the papilla or duct opening. A small wire on a specialized catheter uses electric current to cut the tissue. The actual cut is quite small, usually less than 1/2 inch. This small cut also allows various treatments in the ducts, like stent placement and sweeping of the ducts.

Two cuts can be made. The most common is to the entrance of the bile duct, called a biliary sphincterotomy. Sometimes that is enough to bring relief for the SOD or postcholecystectomy patient. Alternatively, if the biliary sphincterotomy alone does not provide relief, and it is suspected or proven the pancreatic sphincter has high pressures, a cut will be made in both the biliary and pancreatic sphincter.

The most common and serious risk of ERCP is acute pancreatitis, which is severe inflammation of the pancreas. Acute pancreatitis can be deadly. It occurs in up to 30% of the population and is three times more likely to happen if the person is suspected of having SOD as opposed to the general population. Placement of a prophylactic pancreatic duct stent has been shown to limit the incidence of acute pancreatitis as has pre-procedural administration of an indomethacin (NSAID) suppository. If you decide to have an ERCP with sphincterotomy, be sure to ask your doctor if he can include these preventive measures during the procedure.

Other risks with sphincterotomy are bleeding (always tell your doctor what medications you are on, especially those that may interfere with blood clotting), ductal injury, infection, and anything that may arise as a risk factor with anesthesia and an endoscopy.

A somewhat benign side effect of sphincterotomy but worth mentioning is reflux of duodenal contents. This happens because the opening is wider and the sphincter sometimes stays open once it is cut. Rarely, duodenal reflux contents can accumulate in the duct and cause a blockage.

Sphincterotomy commonly needs to be repeated as stenosis, and scar tissue/adhesions can develop in the sphincter area. Stenosis occurs when, over time, the area heals tighter and tighter.

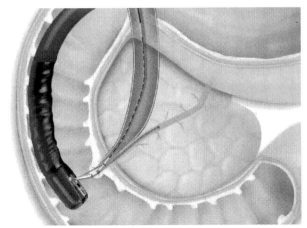

Biliary Sphincterotomy

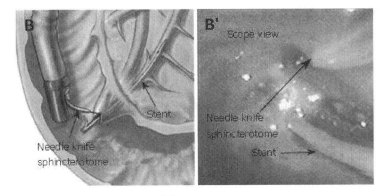

Sphincterotomy

Botox

Botulinum toxin (Botox), a potent inhibitor of acetylcholine release from nerve endings, is injected during an endoscopy procedure. About 50% of patients presenting with postcholecystectomy pain, particularly from SOD, experience symptom relief from this procedure as it reduces basal sphincter pressure. Think of it this way. If someone gets Botox in their forehead, it freezes the muscles so they don't have any forehead lines. The same is true for Botox in the gastrointestinal sphincter area. It freezes the sphincter, preventing it from spasm.

This reduction in pressure may be accompanied by symptom improvement in some patients. For some, Botox is a promising alternative to invasive procedures. The risks of complications are fewer than with most other invasive procedures. The patient is sedated, and the endoscopy tube is sent down the esophagus to the duodenum. There, the Botox is applied.

When risks do arise, they are likely to be associated with either the anesthesia or the Botox itself as an allergy or sensitivity. Other than that, there could be minor side effects related to the placement of the endoscopy tube. Though this is one of the safest procedures, the downside is Botox wears off within a few months and must be repeated, generally, at a minimum of every six months.

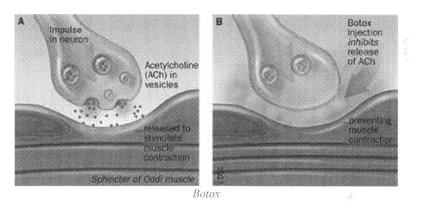

Botox

Celiac Plexus Block

A celiac plexus block is an injection of local anesthetic into or around the celiac plexus of nerves that surrounds the aorta, the main artery in the abdomen. These nerves can carry pain information from the gut or abdominal organ tissues back to the spinal cord and brain. It can be injected into the abdomen, back, or via endoscopic ultrasound (EUS). On occasion, in addition to a local anesthetic, epinephrine, clonidine or a steroid medication may be added to prolong the effects of the celiac plexus block. In extreme cases, the doctor will inject alcohol which will kill the nerve.

Nerve blocks can help relieve postcholecystectomy pain stemming from the biliary area or pancreas. Usually, an anesthesiologist or gastroenterologist will perform this as an outpatient procedure. Most patients receive sedation, so the patient doesn't feel the needle and injection. There is a risk of infection, bleeding, collapsed lung, arterial puncture, nerve damage or drug allergy. There can also be a reaction from the injected medication or from IV sedation or very rarely paralysis. Most commonly, the patient may develop low blood pressure or diarrhea.

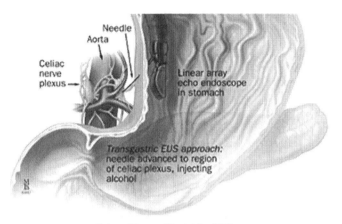

Celiac Plexus Block Via EUS

Spinal Cord Stimulator

A spinal cord stimulator is a medical device surgically implanted under your skin that sends a mild electric current to your spinal cord. A small wire carries the current from a pulse generator to the nerve fibers of the spinal cord. When turned on, the stimulation feels like a mild tingling in the area where the pain is felt. Your pain is reduced because the electrical current interrupts the pain signal from reaching your brain. Stimulation does not eliminate the source of pain, it simply interferes with the signal to the brain, and so the amount of pain relief varies for each person.

A trial period and psychological evaluation are also required to ensure the patient can handle the responsibility of an implantable device, will achieve pain relief, and the stimulation is not unpleasant. The goal for spinal cord stimulation is a 50-70% reduction in pain.

Though this may seem like a miracle device for pain, there are serious risks to consider, including paralysis. Also, the body could form adhesions around the device, which may prevent it from ever being removed. Other risks include infection, bleeding, headache, allergic reaction, spinal fluid leakage, and issues specific to the spinal cord stimulator and lead wires. If your pain is severely affecting your life, this may be a last-resort solution, especially if doctors are completely resistant to prescribing pain medication.

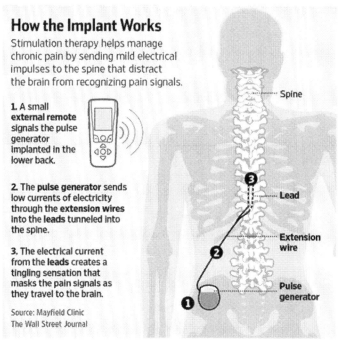

How the Implant Works

Stimulation therapy helps manage chronic pain by sending mild electrical impulses to the spine that distract the brain from recognizing pain signals.

1. A small **external remote** signals the pulse generator implanted in the lower back.

2. The **pulse generator** sends low currents of electricity through the **extension wires** into the **leads** tunneled into the spine.

3. The electrical current from the **leads** creates a tingling sensation that masks the pain signals as they travel to the brain.

Source: Mayfield Clinic
The Wall Street Journal

Spine
Lead
Extension wire
Pulse generator

Spinal Cord Stimulator

Transduodenal Sphincteroplasty

Transduodenal means "through the duodenum." When a doctor performs a sphincteroplasty, he or she slices and sews the sphincter of Oddi, biliary, and/or pancreatic sphincters permanently open. Specific indications for sphincteroplasty include multiple common duct stones or "sludge", primary biliary calculi, unremovable intrahepatic stones, impacted ampullary stones, or stenosis of the sphincter of Oddi.

Gastroenterologists generally do not perform this type of surgery. A surgeon specializing in biliary and pancreatic surgery may perform it as a laparotomy or laparoscopic surgery. Unfortunately, as of this writing, very few surgeons perform this surgery laparoscopically.

I had this surgery as a laparotomy, and it took at least three to four months before I could perform gentle exercises. It was incredibly painful—so painful they had me on ketamine (a horse tranquilizer) and oxymorphone (Dilaudid) intravenously for the pain. Also, the sphincteroplasty opened the floodgates of bile. It was gushing for a few weeks after the surgery. I had a drain coming out of my abdomen that filled constantly. I also had excessive bile diarrhea to the point I had to be on IV fluids around the clock.

These complications did, though, resolve within a month of the surgery. As I said previously, though I experienced complications, I am grateful to have had this surgery.

Transduodenal sphincteroplasty risks include bleeding, infection, and common surgical complications. Rarely will a sphincteroplasty cause acute pancreatitis. Some patients, for unknown reasons, develop chronic pancreatitis after this surgery. I am one of them, though I am uncertain if my chronic pancreatitis was caused by this surgery, medications, years of undiagnosed SOD or previous acute pancreatitis episodes. For some patients, continuing problems and chronic pancreatitis are caused by a "re-stenosis" of the sphincter area and/or accumulation of scar tissue, i.e. adhesions.

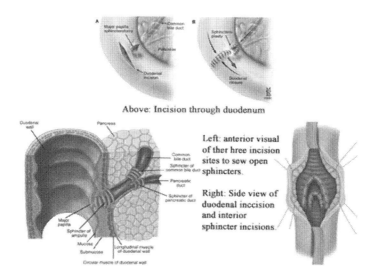

Above: Incision through duodenum

Left: anterior visual of ther hree incision sites to sew open sphincters.

Right: Side view of duodenal inccision and interior sphincter incisions.

Biliary Roux En Y

Biliary roux en y surgery is the nickname for any surgery involving an anastomosis (cutting then reconnecting) of the common bile duct to the duodenum or another cut portion of the small intestine (known as the roux en y limb), diverting it away from the stomach and pancreas. Traditionally, biliary roux en y surgery is indicated for patients with recurrent gallstones requiring repeated intervention, impacted or giant stones, biliary sludge, ampullary stenosis, diseased or cancerous bile duct, dilated lower common bile duct, and restoring continuity to the biliary tract.

Three types of biliary roux en y are choledochoduodenostomy, choledochojejunostomy, and hepaticojejunostomy. They vary in the way the duodenal and/or jejunal portions of the small intestine are reconnected to the bile duct and liver. Your surgeon will determine which procedure will be best for your condition.

Following surgery, the patient's stomach contents (chyme) and pancreatic enzymes continue to empty into the duodenum. As this is occurring, the liver is emptying bile through the bile duct into another area of the small intestine, not the duodenum. The bile will eventually meet up with the chyme and pancreatic enzymes.

Biliary roux en y is major surgery that can be done as a laparotomy or laparoscopically. Recovery time is similar to transduodenal sphincteroplasty surgery. This surgery can cause repeated episodes of cholangitis—a bacterial infection in the bile duct because of translocated bacteria migrating upwards to the jejunal portion of the small intestine, into the bile duct and liver. Other possible complications are hemorrhaging, bile leaks, strictures (narrowing of the bile duct) and any surgery-related complications.

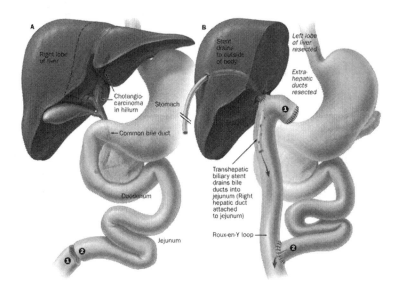

Biliary Roux En Y Example

Feeding Tubes

Since the majority of feeding tubes require a surgical procedure to place them, I figured this was the right chapter to include information on this topic. Feeding tubes won't cure postcholecystectomy syndrome, but they can aid in reducing symptoms and provide nourishment in extreme cases.

The most common feeding tubes for postcholecystectomy patients are the gastrostomyjejunostomy (GJ-tube), which is placed through the stomach, and jejunostomy (J-tube), which is placed through the small intestine. There is also the nasojejunal (NJ-tube), which is a tube threaded from the nose, through the stomach, and into the jejunum. No surgery is required for an NJ tube, but you will have a tube hanging out of your nose rather than your abdomen.

GJ, J, and NJ tubes deliver nutrient-rich liquid formula to the jejunal section of the small intestine, bypassing the stomach, duodenum, sphincter of Oddi area, ducts, and pancreas. In theory, the bile duct, sphincters, and pancreas won't have to do as much work. This, of course, doesn't always happen. All digestive organs can be stimulated instinctually once food enters any part of the body.

I had both GJ and J feeding tubes at different times. They were fraught with complications from the beginning. The first time I had one placed, the pain from the surgical placement was severe, so I stayed in the hospital a few days. The tube kept migrating, and formula would backwash up past the sphincter area and into the stomach, defeating the purpose of the feeding tube. Another time, the tube kinked and I couldn't get the formula to flow. It also took over a month to get the formula right. Add to all this the nuisance of having to hook up to the machine several times a day.

Regardless, though I experienced complications from my feeding tubes and the formula, they served their purpose in helping me gain weight and get much-needed nutrition.

After my sphincteroplasty, I had a peripherally inserted central catheter (PICC) line that delivered total parenteral nutrition (TPN). The PICC line is a central line placed into a large vein usually in the upper arm where liquid nutrition is slowly delivered to the body intravenously. I usually ran it at night to give me freedom during the day. It wasn't so bad, but easily got infected. Showering was a challenge as the lines could not get wet.

I don't know a single person who didn't have issues with feeding tubes and PICC lines. All of them are susceptible to infections, line complications, and can dislodge. However, if you are losing weight at a dangerous rate and can't eat much, one of these alternative nutrition sources may be necessary.

I know very few postcholecystectomy patients who needed a feeding tube or PICC line permanently. Most patients go through short periods of needing them, then bounce back and do fine without them. Those who needed them permanently typically had a comorbid condition like gastroparesis, chronic pancreatitis, or Ehlers-Danlos Syndrome.

GJ and J tubes are usually inserted by a surgeon. PICC lines can be placed by an interventional radiologist. Dieticians, primary care doctors, gastroenterologists, surgeons, and nutritional medical doctors can all manage feeding tube formula and TPN prescriptions. Typically, a visiting nurse will come to your home to help you get started with your feeds and monitor your progress. These services are almost always covered by health insurance. The visiting nurse assigned to me was a doll. I looked forward to her weekly visits and was disappointed when I didn't need the feeding tubes anymore as I missed her company.

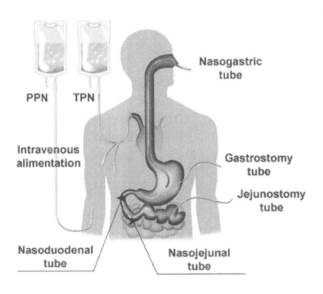

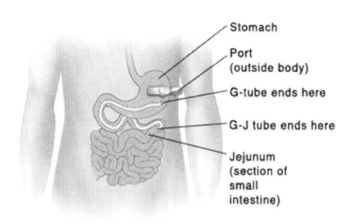

Stomach

Port
(outside body)

G-tube ends here

G-J tube ends here

Jejunum
(section of
small
intestine)

Chapter 8: Be an Empowered Patient

At the beginning of my health journey, I prided myself as a model patient. Whatever I was facing, health-wise, I had faith my doctors would help me. I believed that they believed in me and wanted to help me. I don't doubt every doctor wants the best for their patients. But, over time I learned through pain and misery that not every doctor I consulted was capable of helping me.

I could write dozens of pages about my horrible doctor experiences, but won't. You may already have a long list of negative experiences, so I will spare you. I will say that it became obvious early on that some of my doctors developed opinions of me which impeded their ability to treat me. Others simply did not have the tools or knowledge to help me with postcholecystectomy syndrome. Others were closed-minded to the concept of postcholecystectomy syndrome.

Fortunately, throughout my health journey, I experienced a paradigm shift in my dealings with the medical profession. I went from being a model, meek patient to an empowered, vocal patient advocating for herself.

I wasn't the perfect patient either. One thing I learned about myself was that my expectations of doctors were often unrealistic. If every doctor, nurse, or other healthcare provider is a problem for you, then it's probably your expectations that need to be adjusted and not necessarily the healthcare provider's behaviors that are the problem.

That isn't to say you are in the wrong 100% of the time. I just doubt every single provider was to blame. Even though a large majority of doctors I saw were a complete disappointment, there were a few I cannot say didn't have my best interest in mind. These doctors exhibited compassion and were willing to go the extra mile for me. In addition, they had humility—the ability to admit they didn't know how to help me and made the effort to refer me to another doctor.

At one point in my journey for a diagnosis, I developed a zero-faith attitude toward the healthcare system and its providers. Looking back, I realized many were acting the way they were out of frustration. Here I was, clearly very ill, and yet they, the health professional, could not figure out how to help me.

I had one doctor tell me, "I got into medicine to help people and successfully treat patients. It doesn't seem like you will ever get better, which goes against why I became a doctor." For quite some time, I was infuriated by his comment. In fact, I never saw this doctor again. Today, I understand what he was trying to tell me. His delivery sucked, but I believe he wanted me to be well and just didn't know how to help me.

Possibly, expectations about doctors were engrained in my mind throughout my life. I think most people grow up thinking doctors are God-like. I was no different. I always figured, the rule of life was that I'd go to the doctor if my children or I was sick and my doctor would "fix" us. Usually fixing meant writing a prescription.

When I was severely ill from postcholecystectomy syndrome, I developed an intense anger toward the medical profession when they failed me. How could they not help me? Why were they not believing me? Why were they not doing the legwork to refer me to a doctor who could help me? It was a hopeless and lonely feeling.

I made many mistakes along the way and could write an entire book on how to become an empowered patient. Luckily, there are dozens of these books already written. If you want to read an entire book on becoming an empowered patient, I recommend two books: "The Take-Charge Patient: How You Can Get the Best Medical Care," by Martine Ehrenclou and "The Empowered Patient: How to Get the Right Diagnosis, Buy the Cheapest Drugs, Beat Your Insurance Company, and Get the Best Medical Care Every Time," by Elizabeth S. Cohen. I have read these books and believe every patient should read them.

Finding the Right Doctor

If only there was an online service for patients with postcholecystectomy syndrome matching them with qualified doctors, similar to online dating, life would be much easier. The task of finding the right doctor who will diagnose you can be daunting and frustrating. You may end up having to get a second, third, and even fourth opinion before you get answers to your symptoms.

For those with postcholecystectomy syndrome, you will want to see a gastroenterologist (GI doctor) as their focus is in digestive disorders. I live in a densely-populated region of the U.S. where there are numerous gastroenterology practices from which to choose. I initially chose the practice associated with the emergency room and hospital I frequented for treatment of my postcholecystectomy symptoms. Now I know to research doctors more thoroughly rather than go the route I chose.

In my experience, the best way to learn about a doctor is from other patients. Look at patient review sites on the Internet, which are websites where patients can rate their doctor, usually on a scale of one to five stars. Some include patient comments. Plug the term "doctor rating" into any search engine, and the top doctor rating sites will appear. Some I have used are www.vitals.com, www.healthgrades.com, www.zocdoc.com, and www.ratemds.com. I personally would not see a doctor who had less than a four-star rating on these sites. My health is a life or death matter. I take it very seriously and refuse to have substandard doctors on my care team.

Another way to learn about a doctor is through online support groups and forums for postcholecystectomy syndrome. Other patients can recommend a doctor or steer you away from a horrible doctor. This is how I found the doctor who diagnosed me with SOD. I had to travel halfway across the United States, but it was worth it. On that note, be open to traveling out of town, state or country if your health insurance will permit it.

Call the doctor's practice and ask if they recognize and treat postcholecystectomy syndrome or issues following gallbladder removal. I wouldn't be surprised if most of practices you query are unfamiliar with this syndrome. However, some may have patients who have had difficulty following gallbladder removal.

Don't completely discount a practice that is unfamiliar with postcholecystectomy syndrome. Ask if they are equipped to test for postcholecystectomy conditions like SIBO, SOD, or other uncommon conditions. The more testing the practice offers, the more likely you will obtain the diagnosis and treatment you need.

I cannot impress upon you enough that finding the right doctor is the most important thing you can do. You are already sick. Trust me, if you go to a doctor or several doctors who mistreat you, refuse to validate your symptoms, are not open minded to postcholecystectomy syndrome or aren't equipped to test for most postcholecystectomy conditions, it will make you sicker from the traumatization and prolongation of symptoms.

It Is Ok to Move On and Fire a Doctor

A huge mistake of mine while trying to obtain a diagnosis was relying heavily on my local doctors and their schedules. By the time I traveled to the SOD specialist in Minnesota, where I finally got diagnosed and treated, I had already wasted away to 95 pounds and was profoundly weak and disabled. I spent nearly a year putting all my faith into my local doctors who kept telling me whatever I had would go away on its own or that my symptoms were part of a postpartum syndrome.

I was certain my local doctors would finally fix me and that having to wait long periods in between appointments and tests was standard. Looking back, there were clear signs from the beginning they couldn't or wouldn't fix me, but I felt like I would be a bad patient for jumping ship. How wrong was I!

These doctors thought it was perfectly ok for me to continue waiting months between appointments and tests, though my symptoms and health took a nosedive quickly. I will never wait on doctors again. Please, especially if you are losing weight at a dangerous rate, do NOT waste your time with any doctor who does not treat this as an urgent life-threatening manner. I honestly think they believed I was anorexic or mentally ill. If I had to do over again, after the first few months of getting nowhere locally, I would have traveled to that

SOD specialist in Minnesota much sooner. If he couldn't help me I would have found another doctor and so on.

Most of the doctors I no longer see don't even know I fired them. I just never went back to them. There is no need to inform them of your plans to move on. Simply sign a release so your new doctors can access your medical records. I don't go around firing every doctor who doesn't meet every need. That would be reckless. I do get rid of doctors who have bad bedside manners, aren't compassionate, won't perform testing, are close-minded to alternative treatments, make me wait more than an hour repeatedly, and aren't thorough.

Bring an Advocate

The second mistake I made, next to sticking with bad doctors, was not bringing a good advocate with me to doctor's appointments. With the urgency of my condition, I really needed someone to put their foot down with doctors, especially the GI doctor who could have performed an ERCP right here in my hometown.

My mom accompanied me to most of my appointments and procedures. However, in time, being my mom, advocate, appointment companion, child care provider, etc. became a lot for one person. Regretfully, I should have engaged friends, my adult son, husband at the time, anyone. I needed a natural support system advocating for me at all healthcare appointments.

I noticed that the rare occasions my husband attended doctor appointments with me, doctors listened to him. This was especially true with doctors of certain cultures. It is true that in some cultures, women are to be talked to, not heard from. Sorry, but I wouldn't say it if I hadn't witnessed it firsthand. One local GI doctor who dropped the ball with me did not do the same for male patients I knew.

Worse than not bringing a vocal advocate was going alone to appointments. This proved to be a huge mistake. I was dismissed more readily when I was alone. Also, I had no other witness of conversations that transpired.

Therefore, bring someone, anyone, you know with good advocacy skills. Bring your spouse, parent, adult child, friend, church member, or basically anyone, but don't go alone.

Review Your Doctor's Office Notes and Medical Records

Just as I advised to review your bloodwork, routinely ask for your office notes and medical records from your primary care doctor and all specialist appointments. I decided a year into my health nightmare to acquire and read all my medical records and office notes. It was both a Godsend and a huge let down.

I should have reviewed my health records all along, not a year after my illness. I was shocked to read how many incorrect and defamatory statements were written about me. Reading some of my doctors' office notes was nothing short of eye-opening. In fact, several doctors wrote downright false accounts of my office visit and what transpired.

The tone of some of these doctors and other healthcare providers was nothing short of blaming and shaming the patient for being ill. Unfortunately, I could not do anything about these records as they were a year or two old and, in some cases, I was the only person besides the doctor who participated in my appointment. If you come across anything in your records that is false or derogatory, contact the doctor's practice and request this information be corrected.

Be Strong

I was sick and frightened over my illness to the point I would cry at every office visit. This reaffirmed to the doctors I had mental health issues and not a real disorder. I know it is depressing to be sick and difficult to not cry every time you are in a doctor's office, but try your hardest to pull yourself together.

It is ok to appear sick. You don't want to walk into a doctor's appointment or procedure acting all sunshine and rainbows or have perfect hair and makeup. If you do, I can guarantee your doctor

133

won't see you as an urgent case. Be the sick person you are but try not to cry or at least not that ugly, sobbing cry at every appointment. I literally could feel the growing tension in the air during appointments when I'd be crying. I think it made my doctors uncomfortable.

Anger isn't helpful either. I know it's difficult not to feel anger if you aren't getting help for your condition or if you are treated like a second-class citizen, but try your best to not completely lose your cool. Be assertive but not aggressive, argumentative or combative.

Stand Up for Yourself

I interacted with some wonderful nurses and doctors, but sadly I also experienced downright awful and nasty nurses and doctors at times. Keep in mind, not everyone loves their jobs, and that includes some nurses and doctors. Their attitudes and treatment of you can negatively affect your quality of care and impede your recovery.

It is well-known that the nursing profession has a high burnout rate, and understandably so. The same holds true for some doctors. Burnout is a huge factor with long hours, but some may not even like their jobs. In an online Medscape/WebMD questionnaire of 24,000 doctors representing 25 specialties, only 54%, said they would choose medicine again as a career. 41% would choose the same specialty again. Only a quarter of doctors said they would choose the same practice setting, compared with 50% a year prior.

Why such frustration and discontent among physicians? The survey cited declining incomes, excessive paperwork, and vast uncertainty about changes dictated by the United States Affordable Care Act.

In my opinion, this survey was quite accurate. About half the medical staff I encountered were compassionate, empathetic, caring, interested in my well-being, smart, and thorough. In the hospital setting, resident doctors (doctors who completed medical school and were working on their final residency requirements) were more eager to help me and show compassion. I surmised they hadn't become jaded yet. I wish I could find them now to tell them how wonderful they treated me and to not lose sight of that quality.

Not every emergency room, hospital, or doctor's office experience will be entirely good or entirely bad. My hope for you is regardless of your experience, you will act as an empowered patient and advocate for yourself, not tolerating substandard care. In the event you feel the need to make a formal complaint about a doctor or hospital, follow these suggestions (taken from Trisha Torrey's article, "Complain About a Doctor or Other Healthcare Provider").

Remember that everyone has an occasional bad day. However, a pattern of mistakes, arrogance or misconduct which have resulted in detriment to a patient may mean that doctor or another provider should be reported to someone who can help affect change or remove that provider from practice.

Always begin by complaining directly to the doctor who created the problem. If approaching the doctor directly doesn't get you anywhere, contact the practice manager and make a verbal report, followed by a letter or email that spells out your complaint and your expectations as discussed by phone.

Be aware there will be ramifications if you make a formal complaint and the doctor knows you were the source. If you can find another doctor easily then that is not a big deal. But, if you are looking to preserve your relationship, be mindful a doctor can and will drop you. Patient abandonment is frowned upon but happens all the time.

Do not become that patient who complains about every doctor he or she meets. Doctors talk amongst themselves, and any resistance will be noted in your medical records.

Even if an issue didn't take place in the hospital, find out what hospitals your doctor is affiliated with and complain to two of their personnel: 1. whoever oversees patient relations and 2. whomever oversees risk management. Call the hospital to ask for the names and mailing addresses of the people who hold those positions.

Complain to your local medical society. There is probably not much they can do, but if they begin to see a pattern about one doctor from many sources, they will contact the doctor and try to suggest some sort of correction. Find your local medical society by searching on the Internet for the phrase "medical society" with the name of your city, county or state.

Complain to your doctor's medical board. You can tell which boards those are by searching your doctor online, then finding the information about his training and certifications, such as "Board Certified by _____." You could also call their practice and ask on which boards he or she is certified. Some boards have their own complaint procedures listed on their websites. If the board your doctor was certified by doesn't have a formal complaint procedure, then find an address on the "Contact us" page, and ask that it be delivered to someone who looks at disciplinary or revocation issues.

Complain to the Joint Commission. Hospitals fear The Joint Commission (https://www.jointcommission.org) (formerly called JHACO) and do not want them knocking at their door. The Joint Commission is the organization that accredits hospitals and works toward improved safety for patients, among other hospital quality efforts. If your complaint is associated with an emergency room visit or hospital stay, you can submit a complaint online or in a letter.

Complain to your state's professional licensing bureau, medical board, and/or health or insurance department. Each state handles complaints about medical professionals differently.

Hopefully, you won't ever have to make a verbal or written complaint, but if you do, don't expect miracles to happen, apologies to be made, or acknowledgment of wrong-doing. Practice acceptance around the fact you may never get justice for whatever happened or didn't happen. The point is your complaint could help the next person complaining or something may be done about the problem.

Acknowledge the Good Doctors

Show your appreciation to the doctors who took the time to listen, swiftly acted to diagnose, were open-minded to referring you to another doctor, had compassionate bedside manners, and went the extra mile for you.

Send them a thank you note, a holiday card, and anything to voice your appreciation. If you have a hobby like knitting, woodwork, photography, painting, etc. gift your doctor's practice with something you made. Keep it inexpensive, though. There is no need to spend a lot of money on your homemade gift. They will appreciate the thought, time and effort you spent on making them something.

Chapter 9: Self-Care and Support

You have been through rounds of testing, been jabbed so many times with IV needles you feel like a human pin cushion. You are relieved you have a name for your condition or you still don't know what is causing your postcholecystectomy symptoms. Possibly, you have minor symptoms and have had success utilizing a more natural treatment approach. Or, you may be in remission and are waiting for the proverbial shoe to drop. Whatever has brought you here to read this book, or how severe or benign your symptoms are, it is important you take measures for caring for yourself.

The most important thing is to find your own tried and true self-care tools and put them in an imaginary self-care toolbox. Hence, you will know what to try when things go awry. We are all different and what one person may like or need can be vastly different from the next person.

I like to get facials, pedicures, and massages while someone else may hate to be touched by a stranger. I find meditation and reiki to be very healing while someone else prefers relaxing in a hot bubble bath. I love yoga and hiking, while another person may like to jog, something I have never liked doing. Knitting, crocheting, and watching my favorite television shows soothes me while someone else prefers painting, drawing, or playing a video game.

Take the time to discover yourself or reawaken a long-lost hobby or passion. Even though you may be living with chronic illness and/or pain, it doesn't mean life is over. Anything that can distract from your symptoms is worth exploring.

My first suggestion is to re-read the Natural Treatments chapter again and use it as a reference for ideas on how to naturally keep symptoms at bay. Many of the natural treatments I suggested can be used to achieve emotional balance as well as aid physical symptoms. Look online for self-soothing ideas. There are literally hundreds of ways you can be kind to yourself and self-soothe.

Some patients, including me, find support groups to be therapeutic as meeting other patients can provide a sense of validation and hope. Also, other patients possess a wealth of knowledge for treatments that worked and didn't work.

Support groups

I was relieved when I found my first postcholecystectomy support group online. I was no longer alone. Meeting others like me validated the fact my condition was real even when my doctors were convinced it was psychological. I met others who had the same symptoms and often the exact same experiences with the health care system.

My local doctors consistently treated me as though my symptoms were all in my head. I was starting to wonder if I was indeed losing my mind, that there was no end in sight, no diagnosis, and no treatment to help me. I found it reassuring to meet others with similar symptoms and experiences. It also gave me the opportunity to learn from others. In an online support forum, I found the name of the doctor who ultimately diagnosed me. I learned about natural treatments that helped others. And, I got much-needed support for my feeding tube when I was at a loss of what to do.

You can find support groups on Facebook by putting in the key-words "gallbladder removal" or "postcholecystectomy" in the search field at the top. Groups will appear as suggested pages or groups. Most are the same but with different rules, moderators, and number of group members. Other support groups can be found online by searching Internet search engines. The website www.inspire.com has several digestive disease-specific groups.

If anonymity is a major issue for you, I recommend using a friend's or family member's online account or make up a pseudonym for an online account. Also, you don't have to participate in online support groups to benefit from them. You can simply lurk and read others' posts.

I used the search tool in the Facebook support groups and other online forums to find specific topics I wanted to know about when I didn't want to bother with posting a question or comment. Usually, this field is at the top right or somewhere you can put in a keyword and search through posts. For example, say you are too embarrassed to ask about bile diarrhea. Instead of posting, you can search in the group's search field for "bile diarrhea." The searches generally go back several years so you should be able to see everything anyone ever wrote about bile diarrhea.

One of the benefits of support groups is developing friendships with other patients struggling with postcholecystectomy syndrome. I have support group friends who I've talked with on the phone and even visited in person. There is even a group of us who send holiday greeting cards to each other. Some support group members have helped me through the worst days—as much as my family or "healthy" friends because they could relate. I feel safe with my online friends and know they have my back whenever I need them. Some are like sisters to me.

My friend Kelly has been the greatest blessing. She somehow found me on a support group forum and sent me an email asking about my experience with the pancreatic enzyme, Creon. I don't know how it all happened, but we became the best of friends. Though much of our friendship has been via email and phone as she lives on the west coast while I live on the east coast, we make a point to meet up in New York City once a year. Recently, I traveled to visit her at her home on the west coast. She has been my biggest supporter and cheerleader.

Although support groups can be helpful for some people, for others they can make matters worse. Many people who frequent chronic illness support groups are in the throes of illness and pain. Keep in mind, when people experience remission or freedom from symptoms the last place they will likely visit is a support group. Instead, they will be out living their lives and making up for lost time from when they were ill. A few of us stick around to give back and offer support and hope, but we are few and far between. It is unfortunate when people who are doing well leave support groups as it can seem dismal and hopeless if you are in a support group with no healthy people.

A friend of mine who was experiencing mysterious postcholecystectomy symptoms joined a Facebook support group I had suggested. I thought it would help her get support, so she didn't feel so alone with her symptoms. Well, she ended up fleeing the group just as soon as I added her. The stories of people suffering and the length of time they suffered was frightening for her. She is doing well today and ended up benefiting from natural treatments. I completely understood, and it got me to thinking how unfortunate it is that so many people don't stick around to show people there is hope and to just hang in there.

Mental Health Therapy

Anyone with a chronic health condition, especially one that is unexplained, will likely experience some depression and anxiety regardless of how strong their mental health was prior to their illness. When my symptoms were at their worst, I'd cry day and night and experienced crippling anxiety

My chronic illness and pain were often too much to bear. Regretfully, I didn't seek mental health treatment, outside of medications until after the worst of my symptoms resolved. I should have sought help sooner. Instead, I waited until the health crisis was over. Seeking mental health treatment is important as poor mental health status has been known to exacerbate health conditions and contribute to poor health outcomes.

By the time I recuperated from my health crisis, I had developed an intense fear and resentment of doctors and hospitals. Over the past few years, I've had several severe pancreatic pain episodes, yet I refused to go to the emergency room because of my health-related post-traumatic stress disorder (PTSD).

There were many contributing factors to my PTSD, including mistreatment by health care staff, doctors not believing me, being treated as a drug seeker because of normal test results, isolation from

141

society, nearly dying, spending a good portion of a year in the hospital, having to be hooked up to a feeding tube every day, all the IVs stuck in me to the point I have one good arm vein left for blood draws, and the fact I was sick around the clock for several years.

It is not uncommon to experience health-related PTSD. Some patients develop a fear of doctors and hospitals, a fear of eating, and a fear of illness in general. Some avoid doing things they used to enjoy for fear it will cause a flare up. Others experience frustration from loved ones and feel alone and isolated.

A therapist once told me that the form of PTSD I had from my health nightmare was akin to those coming back from war or patients who survived stage 4 cancer. I say that not to downplay the severity of those types of PTSD. Instead, never underestimate the damage postcholecystectomy syndrome can do to one's mental, emotional, and spiritual state.

If you have had perfect care from doctors and healthcare staff, limited exposure to hospitals, and experienced minimal symptoms, then possibly you cannot relate to how bad it could possibly be. If this is the case, kudos to you and count yourself very fortunate. I have met many patients who get diagnosed immediately, find treatments that work, and have compassionate doctors. Their condition has very little effect on their mental state. For those who don't have this experience, therapy may be warranted.

The best form of therapy I received was from a licensed social worker who was also a hypnotherapist. He helped teach me coping and self-soothing skills not only for my pain but also for the mental anguish I endured, which was an entirely different type of pain. He also incorporated evidenced-based trauma treatment techniques.

There are many different types of mental health therapy. I personally would only see a therapist trained in at least one evidence-based modality. Some of the most common therapies for trauma are Cognitive Behavioral Therapy (CBT), Narrative Exposure, Prolonged Exposure, and Eye Movement Desensitization and

Reprocessing (EMDR). Most psychotherapists are versed in CBT, also known as "Talk Therapy."

I experienced positive results with CBT, which focuses on exploring relationships among a person's thoughts, feelings, and behaviors. During CBT, a therapist will actively work with a patient to uncover unhealthy patterns of thought and how they may be causing self-destructive behaviors and beliefs. CBT helps you become aware of inaccurate or negative thinking so you can view challenging situations more clearly and respond to them in a more effective way.

CBT can be a very helpful tool in treating mental health disorders, such as depression, PTSD, or an eating disorder. However, not everyone who benefits from CBT has a mental health condition. It can be an effective tool to help anyone learn how to better manage stressful life situations.

I have heard great things about EMDR, a psychotherapy treatment that was originally designed to alleviate the distress associated with traumatic memory. According to the EMDR Humanitarian Assistance Programs website, EMDR therapy is an eight-phase treatment which comprehensively identifies and addresses experiences that have overwhelmed the brain's natural resilience or coping capacity, and have thereby generated traumatic symptoms and/or harmful coping strategies. Through EMDR therapy, patients can reprocess traumatic information until it is no longer psychologically disruptive.

Psychopharmacology (psychiatric medication) is also an effective way to treat anxiety, depression and/or trauma. However, it is well-documented that psychopharmacology alone is not as beneficial as combining it with psychotherapy. In other words, popping a pill and expecting a miracle isn't the best way to deal with mental health issues. Popping a pill and regularly seeing a therapist is more evidence-based and will produce better outcomes.

There are many different types of psychiatric medications, including antidepressants, antipsychotics, mood stabilizers and anti-anxiety medications. In my opinion and experience, do not rely on your family physician to prescribe these medications. Go to a psychiatric nurse practitioner or psychiatrist. These individuals are well-versed in what works best for each person's situation and body chemistry. An added benefit is some psychiatric medications have a positive effect on certain gastrointestinal conditions.

Ask about genetic testing to see which medications to try and which to avoid for your genetic body type. Since these medications are heavily metabolized by the liver's cytochrome P450 pathway, genetic mutations of this pathway's liver enzymes can predict which psychiatric medications will work best for you.

If you want to steer clear of pharmaceuticals, you could stick with talk therapy or seek a consult with a natural health practitioner. He or she may be able to treat your condition with supplements, herbs, or diet. There are many ways to tackle anxiety and depression with natural treatments.

Spiritual Support

Whether you are an atheist, agnostic or deeply religious person, strengthening your spiritual condition will most certainly benefit you. For atheists or agnostics, you may feel spiritual by taking the time to be with nature or quieting the mind through meditation. If you are religious or have a devotion to a religion or school of thought, think about increasing your attendance and presence at your religion's or spiritual practice's gathering place.

Get involved in prayer or spiritual study groups and let people know you need prayers. I firmly believe the power of prayer contributed to me getting well again. I had so many people praying for me— friends, family, and even strangers on Facebook. I don't know how to describe it other than I "felt" the love and now that I am better, believe prayers helped me.

If you are too sick or exhausted to leave the house, you can watch religious or spiritual services online. You'd be surprised how many different types of religious services you can attend right from the comfort of your own couch or bed. Some worldwide churches have cell phone apps to watch services and deliver special messages. I have satellite radio in my car and have used it to listen to the religious/spiritual channels. Also, uplifting podcasts, both religious and spiritual, can be accessed through your phone or computer.

Pick up a devotional daily meditation book that is religious or spiritual. You can also find these geared specifically for people with chronic pain and illness. The most important thing is that you find something that will reinforce positive messages and an attitude of faith and hope. I find starting my day off reading a daily meditation from my spiritual practice starts the day off much better than when I neglect to read it.

Something else to consider is Chronic Pain Anonymous. It is a wonderful 12-step spiritual, not religious program, for people with chronic pain and chronic illness. There aren't many face-to-face in-person meetings, but they have at least one phone or online meeting every day. Their website is www.chronicpainanonymous.com. Through the therapeutic value of support and the 12 steps (adopted from programs like Alcoholics Anonymous and Narcotics Anonymous), you can learn to cope and live with chronic pain and chronic illness. The cornerstone of 12-step programs like this is "working" spiritual principles like surrender, open-mindedness, acceptance, honesty, and willingness.

Journaling

University of Texas at Austin psychologist and researcher James Pennebaker contends that regular journaling strengthens immune cells, called T-lymphocytes. Pennebaker believes that writing about stressful events helps you come to terms with them, thus reducing the impact of these stressors on your physical health. One study showed that daily journaling decreased the symptoms of asthma and rheumatoid arthritis.

Psych Central lists the following benefits of journaling:

Clarify your thoughts and feelings. Do you ever seem all jumbled up inside, unsure of what you want or feel? Taking a few minutes to jot down your thoughts and emotions (no editing!) will quickly get you in touch with your internal world.

Know yourself better. By writing routinely you will get to know what makes you feel happy and confident. You will also become clear about situations and people who are toxic for you—important information for your emotional well-being.

Reduce stress. Writing about anger, sadness, and other painful emotions helps to release the intensity of these feelings. By doing so, you will feel calmer and better able to stay in the present.

Solve problems more effectively. Typically, we problem solve from a left-brained, analytical perspective. But sometimes the answer can only be found by engaging right-brained creativity and intuition. Writing unlocks these other capabilities and affords the opportunity for unexpected solutions to seemingly unsolvable problems.

Resolve disagreements with others. Writing about misunderstandings rather than stewing over them will help you to understand another's point of view. And you just may come up with a sensible resolution to the conflict.

Journaling has been a cathartic way for me to visually get my feelings out and articulate my needs and wants. Frequently, I felt like people were sick of hearing me whine about my illness. Writing provided a safe venue to vent, even if I was the only person reading it. I also like that I can go back a few years and see the evidence of how far I've come.

Music Therapy

Listening to music can be inspiring, motivating, and relaxing. Depending on my mood, I'll listen to anything from hip-hop to classical music. According to the American Music Therapy Association, music can be a powerful and physically noninvasive medium for improving pain and chronic illness.

Music Therapy is an established health profession in which music is used within a therapeutic relationship to address physical, emotional, cognitive, and social needs of individuals. Music Therapy is the clinical and evidence-based use of music interventions to accomplish individualized goals within a therapeutic relationship by a credentialed professional who has completed an approved music therapy program.

I've never participated in a music therapy session. However, music is a very important part of my daily recovery practice. If I want to relax, I'll listen to soft, easy music. If I need some inspiration, I'll listen to upbeat, positive music. If I need to get rid of rage, I'll listen to heavy metal or angry rap music.

I've adopted a few go-to theme songs that are my own personal anthems. Your personal theme songs will be songs that inspire you, leaving you filled with hope and faith. I like Rachel Platton's "Fight Song", Tim McGraw's "Live Like You Were Dying", and Kelly Clarkson's "Stronger". After my husband left me, Pink's "So What", Destiny Child's "Survivor", and Gloria Gaynor's "I Will Survive", were very helpful.

Stay away from sad, depressing songs.

Stop Going to Doctors

At some point, frequent doctor visits may be doing you more harm than good. If all you are doing in your spare time is going to doctors and hospitals, obsessing over a diagnosis and cure, and going bankrupt because of high co-pays, consider taking a short break from it all.

Obviously, if you need to head to the emergency room, do it. But, consider a break from the healthcare system if you are exhausted like I was from constantly seeing doctors, most of whom were unable to help me.

I experienced some moments of wellness and peace of mind when I stuck to natural health practitioners and natural remedies, stayed off the Internet, and rescheduled all my specialist appointments for a month or two later. During this time, I spent time with family, rested, meditated, treated myself to pedicures and manicures, started crocheting and knitting, binge-watched television shows, and worked on my first book.

It was as if I took a vacation from being sick and, most importantly, from worrying about being sick and getting pissed off at doctors. Obviously, at some point, I had no choice but to see my doctors, but the respite from all things medical was lovely.

Dealing with Financial Implications

Many postcholecystectomy patients continue to work and excel in their career field. For 13 years, I climbed the ranks of a statewide advocacy organization, earning several promotions and recognition as a national expert in children's mental health and juvenile justice practices. The entire time I had postcholecystectomy syndrome. I attended conferences and ate at restaurants with funders and policymakers but too often retreated to my hotel room in pain. Regardless, I learned to live with it and refused to allow my symptoms to get in the way of my career.

God was definitely on my side when I changed jobs in 2010. My new employer offered a long-term disability plan which I could have cared less about at the time of my hire. Though I had postcholecystectomy symptoms, I was healthy and never thought I would need it. Boy, was I wrong.

In May 2012, after nine months of barely keeping it together at work because of the severity of my symptoms, I had to take a leave of absence. By August 2012, I could comfortably leave my position thanks to that long-term disability policy, which enabled me to collect 60% of my income. The insurance company then forced me to apply for social security disability so they could collect their share. I received it on my first try.

I strongly encourage anyone with mild symptoms to get a long-term disability policy as soon as possible. Do not hesitate. See if you can get one—no matter what the cost—that will pay out for pre-existing conditions. Contact your human resources department to see if they offer such a policy through your employer or search online for insurance companies that offer it. It is well worth the cost of the premium.

If you are currently unable to work and live in the United States, consult with a social security disability attorney. Let them do the work of getting you qualified. The key to social security or any disability program is to have the support of your doctors. I scheduled office appointments with my physicians specifically to complete the forms required to document that I was disabled and unable to work. Do not think your doctors will complete these forms just because they received them. Not one of my doctors voluntarily completed these forms. I had to persist. My primary care doctor and his staff have been amazing with getting documents submitted. However, the specialists required extra nudging.

When it is time to enroll in a health care plan at work, be sure to pick the best plan for inpatient and emergency room copays. During the year my illness landed me in the hospital repeatedly, my health insurance's inpatient copay was $1,000. I was in the hospital at least ten times, so do the math. Another year, we had a plan where I had to pay a copay for everything—every blood draw, scan, imaging study, procedure, etc. I had bill collectors sending notices and, by working out a payment plan, I was able to settle my mounting health debt.

Some patients say that work and their careers kept them going through the worst symptom experiences. Others claim working made their symptoms worse. Whatever the case, explore all financial options that can support you when you need to heal and recover. Be prepared for the worst even if it never happens.

If you live in the United States, utilize the Family Medical Leave Act (FMLA) to take short leaves of absence from your job. FMLA does not ensure you will get paid during that time but is meant to protect you from losing your job. Caregivers can apply for FMLA as well if they need to care for you.

149

Be Kind to Yourself

I had to learn to be kind to myself throughout my illness. I had to stop saying horrible things about myself to myself that I would never think of saying to another person. I'd get in a sickness rut and tell myself I was a loser, terrible wife and mother, hopeless, ugly, etc. I had to put post-it notes around my house telling me I would be ok, that I was a good person and other positive affirmations. I read a great book called, "The Anatomy of Hope," about people dealing with chronic illness who never gave up hope no matter how grim their circumstances. I recommend reading it.

I had to quit weighing myself on my bathroom scale. I'd obsess over my drastic weight loss, weighing myself several times a day, driving myself crazy if I lost a pound. The fear of wasting away was awful. The actual wasting away was awful too. I was so thin I despised the way I looked.

It took a while, but I eventually stopped obsessively weighing myself, found clothes that flattered my shrinking body, and developed acceptance around my situation and appearance. I admit a small part of me still fears losing weight again, though I now weigh the most I ever have.

Possibly, you have had the opposite side effect of having your gallbladder removed and have gained weight. Regardless, having to purchase clothes due to weight fluctuations can get costly. I quickly learned to rely heavily on thrift stores and friends' hand me downs. You would not believe the deals I found and the designer clothes people donated to places like the Salvation Army and Goodwill. I once found a pair of designer Miss Me jeans worth $120.00 for $3.99!

Therefore, for erratic weight loss and weight gain, hit the local thrift store. Ebay has some good deals too. Or, let your friends know you need clothing donations. Since most of my friends were bigger than my tiny frame, I accepted donations from their teenage and college-age daughters and ended up looking quite hip in American Eagle, Hollister, and Abercrombie and Fitch brands of clothing.

Another way you can be kind to yourself is to stay off Internet health sites. I was obsessed with trying to figure out what was wrong with me to the point I couldn't stop searching the Internet. Although doing Internet research helped me get better and enabled me to write this book, I often went incredibly overboard with the amount of time I spent online, something my mom routinely commented on. Limit the time you spend online and stick to it! Spending an entire day on the Internet is not necessary and will only frustrate and scare you. Additionally, not all the information you read online is factual.

Watch your television viewing time too. The television became both my best friend and my enemy, depending on the day and my mood. I was couch- and bed-bound for so long that I ran out of things to watch. I can't believe some of the trash I watched. The worst were reality or talk shows where everyone looked perfect and had really stupid problems (in comparison to my life-threatening problems).

Luckily, I figured out that I needed comedy in my life and forced myself to watch comedies—any comedy television show or movie—until I found something that made me laugh. Laughter truly can be the best medicine.

Instead of watching too much television, I'd read, play a computer game, and took up hobbies. Walk into any craft store, and you will find an endless array of hobby items and kits to purchase, ex. jewelry making kits, calligraphy, needlepoint, scrapbooking, painting, drawing, and weaving.

While I was sick, I started knitting and crocheting again and am so glad I did. Making crocheted and knitted items has become a great way to give back to people who have helped me. I've even made things for my doctors and their nursing staff. Another hobby I took up that has become popular is adult coloring books. They have great designs and patterns to choose from. You can use crayons, markers, or colored pencils.

Stick with Positive People

My family did whatever they could to support and comfort me. Friends, however, came and went. I had to routinely examine friendships. For the most part, I had supportive friends who stuck by my side. Some couldn't deal with my illness or just went on with their busy lives. I am glad they showed this trait as I realized the hard way how valuable good, faithful friends were. I don't need unsupportive people in my life, and neither do you.

Recognize that some losses end up being a good thing. For example, I met a woman who went through a horrible time with severe postcholecystectomy symptoms, ERCPs, and surgery. Her husband cheated on her and abandoned her only a few months after she had major surgery. It was painful to hear. But, the good news was that his leaving was a positive thing. She recovered from her postcholecystectomy issues, healed emotionally, and is now in a much better, loving relationship. I can say the same about my own marriage. At the time my husband left, I thought it was the end of the world. Today, I am the happiest I've been in many years.

Set boundaries with toxic people. Obviously, for some of you this will be difficult as the toxic person could be your spouse, child, other close family member or lifelong friend. I am not saying you need to divorce your husband or wife or disown family members and friends. Instead, learn to set healthy boundaries with the help of a therapist or attend Al-anon if the toxic person is an addict or alcoholic. Focus on spending most of your time with positive and supportive people.

For Caregivers, Family, and Friends

For those of you reading this book as a caregiver, friend, or family member of a postcholecystectomy patient, thank you for hanging in there. I know it isn't easy and, at times, can be overwhelming. My heart goes out to you.

You may wonder how you can be most helpful to someone with postcholecystectomy syndrome. Being a nonjudgmental supporter is the best thing you can offer this person. Validate his or her symptoms and ask how you can help them through this difficult time. If they have a hard time asking for help, offer to run an errand, watch a child, accompany him or her to a doctor's appointment or procedure (this is by far one of the most helpful things you can do), or cook a meal they can actually eat. Anything that takes stress off him or her is helpful.

Some patients need someone to be their voice at doctor's appointments and emergency room visits as not all medical professionals understand or know about postcholecystectomy syndrome. Having an advocate on board boosts a patient's chances of getting adequate treatment. Insist on attending appointments and procedures with your loved one.

If you play a significant role as a caregiver, be sure to take care of yourself. It can be frustrating and oftentimes depressing to be the caregiver of a person with severe postcholecystectomy syndrome. My soon-to-be husband and entire family were saints throughout my health nightmare. The best thing I could do as the sick person was push them to do fun things even if I had to stay home. They had every right to enjoy life. Caregivers shouldn't be expected to stay home every time we do. Sometimes pushing myself to do things with my husband, kids, friends, or family was the best gift I could give them. I didn't have to be on top of my game. I just needed to be there.

Caregivers can also try creative ways to bring happiness and fun to the patient stuck in bed or on the couch. Watch a movie together. Read a book or magazine to them. Listen to an audio book together. Play a board or card game. Color or paint together. Do a jigsaw puzzle. The possibilities are endless.

Chapter 10: No Diagnosis, No Treatment: What to Do/What Could It Be?

If you are the unfortunate patient who has endured extensive testing and trialed countless treatments, yet still do not have a diagnosis or feel better, you aren't alone. It isn't uncommon for postcholecystectomy patients to have normal bloodwork and scans. Sadly, though, postcholecystectomy syndrome continues to go unnoticed in research circles and by the medical profession. Therefore, consider yourself an enigma.

Rather than removing so many gallbladders, the medical profession needs to put forth the effort to find alternative ways to retain the gallbladder in most patients. This would essentially eliminate postcholecystectomy syndrome altogether. Naturally, in some cases, gallbladder surgery will be unavoidable, no matter what alternative and preventative treatments are employed.

Since I do not foresee the medical profession limiting gallbladder surgery anytime soon, it is imperative researchers work on investigating the origins of postcholecystectomy syndrome and conduct clinical trials to resolve symptoms. Instead, research is focused on specific diseases that have a name. Postcholecystectomy syndrome is a blanket term for any condition resulting from gallbladder removal; and, as such, very little attention is paid to this elusive condition.

This is not only frustrating to the patient, but also to medical professionals wanting to help their patients feel better. Hopefully, in time, postcholecystectomy syndrome will be more widely recognized, and research associated with this condition will increase.

Till then, lack of research and treatments aren't helping your situation. What you can do is try the treatments listed in this book and take the focus off a diagnosis. It is also quite possible you have a condition not commonly recognized by all doctors or one that is easily diagnosed. You may even have a condition that isn't even associated with your cholecystectomy.

The Most Elusive Conditions

There is an actual condition called Medically Unexplained Physical Symptoms (MUPS). Fibromyalgia and Chronic Fatigue Syndrome used to be MUPS before they had names. Your postcholecystectomy symptoms may fall under MUPS, or you may have an actual condition with a name attached to it.

Regardless, the important thing is to take care of yourself and never give up searching for relief from your symptoms. Yes, it is beneficial to have a clear, definitive diagnosis, but that doesn't mean you cannot work with your doctor or natural health practitioner to find treatments to alleviate your symptoms.

Some postcholecystectomy conditions are certainly easier to diagnose than others. For example, if you experience diarrhea and it is resolved with cholestyramine, you undoubtedly have bile malabsorption or bile acid diarrhea.

Surgical errors can typically be seen on scans. Ulcers, bile reflux, and esophageal conditions can be diagnosed through an endoscopy scope. Most colon conditions can be diagnosed via a colonoscopy. And, many liver and pancreatic conditions can be diagnosed through bloodwork or scans.

However, there are elusive conditions, which are not only difficult to diagnose, but difficult to find a doctor knowledgeable about them. The following are the most difficult-to-diagnose, elusive conditions that could be the cause of your postcholecystectomy symptoms.

Sphincter of Oddi Dysfunction (SOD): SOD is a condition where the sphincter valves controlling the flow of bile and pancreatic fluids do not open and close properly. Ideally, your sphincters (biliary, pancreatic, and Oddi) will open and close in a symbiotic manner.

When a patient has SOD, these sphincters typically spasm shut when they should open. Alternatively, your sphincters could be out of sync

155

and not opening exactly when they should, i.e. the biliary, pancreatic, and Oddi sphincters dysfunction at the same time.

Sphincter dysregulation and sphincters that spasm shut a little too much, not opening when they should, are extremely difficult conditions to diagnose. Elevated liver function results and a dilated bile duct may reveal an SOD condition, but typically, an ERPC with manometry is required.

Medications and natural treatments can help, but sometimes a sphincterotomy or surgery is needed. Locating a doctor well-versed in SOD is a challenge. However, a list of SOD doctors can be found at www.sodae.org.

Biliary colic/spasm: Just like any muscle in the body, the bile duct can spasm, causing pain. People suffering from this condition generally get substantial relief from stents. Stents can control painful spasms and open the bile duct for bile to flow better. Antispasmodic and muscle relaxant medications, particularly long acting, help some people too. The only way of knowing whether this is the cause of your symptoms is by trialing treatments to see if they help your symptoms. Diagnosis is one of excluding other conditions and trialing medications or stents.

Biliary sludge: Bile is a liquid that shouldn't be thick and clumpy. Sludge is bile that contains microscopic gallstone crystals and, due to its thick consistency, doesn't flow freely. Biliary sludge will produce unpleasant symptoms. I think anyone having an ERCP should ask their doctors to collect some bile and have it sent to a lab (rarely ever happens). There, the lab can look at it under a microscope to see if it indeed has gallstone crystals. They can also test to see if the bile is infected with bacteria.

I am quite fond of theories by a Russian doctor named Dr. Turumin. For biliary sludge and postcholecystectomy syndrome, he promotes the use of Celecoxib (Celebrex) and Ursodeoxycholic acid (Ursodiol, Actigall) based on studies he conducted of postcholecystectomy patients. Stents may be helpful too, but can get clogged rather quickly. Plastic stents are more apt to get clogged as opposed to metal cage stents.

Papillary stenosis: Narrowing around the sphincter of Oddi can be triggered by trauma and inflammation due to pancreatitis, instrumentation (ex. ERCP), or prior passage of a stone. People who have had a successful sphincterotomy can experience stenosis with or without scar tissue months or years after the procedure. Treatment is balloon dilatation or repeated sphincterotomy via ERCP. And ERCP and even an endoscopy can detect scar tissue in this area of the body.

Motility Disorders: Anytime there is an assault on the digestive system, i.e. surgery, viruses, hormones, bacteria, fluid change, etc. our regulated digestive system can be thrown off. Depending on how sensitive a person is, even a slight change can result in disabling symptoms. Gastroparesis is an example of a motility disorder typically diagnosed by a gastric emptying study, though not always reliable. Motility issues of the bowel aren't easily diagnosed either unless a bowel motility medication resolves symptoms.

Regarding motility and nausea, as I mentioned in the medications chapter, domperidone helped me. A gastroparesis diet can be helpful as well. There is an excellent book called, "Living Well with Gastroparesis" by Crystal Zaborowski Saltrelli, which I highly recommend.

For bowel motility issues, medications for IBS may resolve symptoms. I also recommend seeking a consult with a functional or Chinese medicine practitioner to "realign" your body and trial natural treatments.

Bile reflux: Stagnant motility of the upper small intestine can result in bile refluxing into the stomach as can a problem with the stomach's pyloric valve, the valve that controls the emptying of stomach contents into the small intestine. Bile acids present in the stomach or esophagus can cause severe pain and nausea. It is difficult diagnosing bile reflux unless, upon endoscopy, there is a copious amount of bile present in the stomach and/or the esophageal tissue is damaged from the bile.

A friend of mine with severe bile reflux gets relief from a combination of domperidone and sucralfate, an acid reducer. Some benefit from taking a bile acid sequestrant that will bind to the bile and sweep it out. Sleeping upright or at an angle can keep bile down. A bed wedge is great for that.

Pancreatic Issues: The pancreas can be an incredibly sensitive organ. Depending on the patient, even a touch of chronic pancreatitis can cause moderate to severe pain, nausea, and loose stools that are sometimes yellow. It can be difficult diagnosing pancreatic conditions as the patient may present with normal bloodwork, scans, and pancreatic functioning tests. Typically, pancreatic enzyme levels will be elevated in bloodwork. However, I and many others have experienced severe flare ups with no elevation in enzyme levels. This is often referred to as minimal change pancreatitis.

There are countless silent and invisible causes to chronic pancreatic inflammation, also known as idiopathic chronic pancreatitis. Idiopathic causes can be from medications, biliary issues, autoimmune disorders, duct strictures, and hereditary or genetic predispositions. Patients with mild chronic pancreatitis may have normal bloodwork, scans, and functional tests. Prescription enzymes and dietary modifications can help along with pain management techniques.

Medications: I can't tell you how many times I've had unexplained digestive or other symptoms, then stopped a medication, and the symptoms completely abated. I've experienced pharmacists and doctors telling me a medicine I was taking couldn't possibly be the cause of a symptom I had, yet it did.

There is no reason you couldn't be that patient who has a rare side effect from a drug. Benzodiazepine, antibiotic, opioid, psychiatric and other medications all have the potential for producing digestive symptoms.

I've also experienced digestive symptoms upon withdrawal of a medication, especially antidepressants and benzodiazepines. Cessation of a medication can also cause severe side effects. There are many medications that cause a withdrawal syndrome, not just addictive medications. Yes, medications and discontinuation of medications *can* cause symptoms mimicking postcholecystectomy syndrome.

Hormonal Dysfunction: As I discussed in Chapter 5, I don't think it is a coincidence most SOD sufferers are women who had their gallbladders removed. The primary hormonal differences between men and women are the reproductive hormones, estrogens, and androgens (ex. testosterone). Estrogens have a profound effect on the gastrointestinal system, androgens not so much. Variations in these hormones not only affect the male and female reproductive system, but also the digestive system and digestive hormones. Men and women have the same hormones, yet there are variations in hormone levels and patterns; and there are differences in how the hormones interact with male and female bodies.

While estrogens are present in both men and women, they are usually present at significantly higher levels in women of reproductive age. Probably the most obvious effect women's hormones have on the digestive system is estrogen's effect on the gallbladder as it regulates CCK hormone and induces a relaxation of CCK-induced tension.

Women are twice as likely as men to have gallstones because estrogen raises cholesterol levels in the bile and slows gallbladder movement. One study on prairie dogs showed that sphincter of Oddi motility was relaxed during estrogen infusion.

Progesterone is another predominantly female hormone which significantly affects gallbladder emptying in response to the CCK hormone by inducing a concentration-dependent relaxation of the gallbladder and alters partitioning of hepatic bile between the gallbladder and small intestine and, therefore, gallbladder filling. In pregnancy, an increase in the hormone progesterone contributes to constipation by slowing the motility of intestinal contractions that

159

move food down the digestive tract. In addition, progesterone causes the stomach's esophageal valve to relax, which could contribute to Gastroesophageal reflux disease (GERD).

The imbalances of estrogen and progesterone can influence the movement of food through the intestines—some by speeding the process up, causing diarrhea, nausea, and abdominal pain; and others by slowing things down and causing bloating and constipation. Therefore, it's probably a good idea to access hormone testing from a functional medicine practitioner or naturopath. I don't recommend hormone testing from a gynecologist unless their expertise is in bioidentical hormone treatment. Gynecologists typically use blood tests that don't provide an accurate view of your hormone status.

HPA axis dysfunction: The hypothalamic–pituitary–adrenal (HPA) axis is the system that makes sure our adrenal glands function correctly, which in turn affects our digestive system. The ultimate result of the HPA axis is to increase levels of cortisol in the blood during times of stress. Cortisol releases glucose into the bloodstream and suppresses and modulates the immune system, digestive system, and reproductive systems.

It has been proven time and again that stress can contribute to digestive issues. Research has shown that HPA dysregulation influences symptoms in irritable bowel syndrome (IBS).

An endocrinologist or primary care physician can order HPA-axis-specific bloodwork. However, conventional testing is generally useless unless your adrenals are in complete failure or you have a pituitary condition. A functional medicine practitioner or naturopath can conduct a saliva cortisol/DHEA test to gauge cortisol readings throughout a given day.

Things that help keep this system in balance are: avoiding sugar and processed foods, gentle exercise—not too much and not too little, avoiding stress, meditation, adrenal supplements, and adequate sleep.

Bacterial Dysbiosis: So many postcholecystectomy patients report experiencing a flare up of symptoms after they have taken a round of antibiotics. In fact, some antibiotics can cause pancreatitis. They can also cause a rebound overgrowth, i.e. SIBO.

Bacteria control every aspect of digestion. If your gut's bacteria are imbalanced, your digestion will be as well. SIBO testing from a gastroenterologist or functional medicine practitioner is helpful for diagnosing bacterial dysbiosis, but is not foolproof. Treatments for this include more antibiotics, herbs, and dietary modifications.

Alternatively, antibiotics can wipe out your gut's good bacteria, which is required for proper digestion. Replenishing your gut with good bacteria found in yogurt, kefir, and probiotics can help get you back on track. Practicing a clean diet can be helpful as well.

Food Intolerance: This is not to be confused with a food allergy. A food intolerance can cause many different symptoms or reactions and can be temporary or lifelong. As described in the diet chapter, keep a diligent food diary for several weeks by recording everything you drank and ate, supplements and medications you took, and activities like exercise. This should reveal an intolerance to a food or beverage.

Dairy can be a big offender due to its lactose content. The proteins in dairy, casein, and whey, can also cause sensitivities. In addition to dairy, gluten can cause problems. Not all celiac disease patients have abnormal bloodwork or endoscopy biopsies. If you or your doctor suspect celiac disease or gluten sensitivity could be to blame for your symptoms, try a gluten free diet.

Microscopic Colitis: Microscopic colitis is an inflammation of the colon that can only be seen with a microscope. Microscopic colitis is a type of inflammatory bowel disease. There are two types of microscopic colitis—collagenous colitis and lymphocytic colitis. Both produce the same symptoms. Causes include autoimmune diseases, medications, infections, genetic factors, and bile acid malabsorption. Symptoms are a strong urgency to defecate, diarrhea, abdominal pain, weight loss, bloating, and/or nausea.

Testing for microscopic colitis is not performed by all gastroenterologists, though it is simply a biopsy performed during colonoscopy. Hopefully, in time, all doctors performing a colonoscopy will be able to test for this condition. Treatments include dietary changes, removal of offending medications, anti-diarrheals, immunomodulators, low dose naltrexone, and steroids.

Nerve/Rib Issue: If your only symptom is pain, it could be caused by a nerve or rib issue, which is difficult to diagnose. If it is a nerve issue you will likely see an improvement in pain with nerve blocks or common nerve medications like gabapentin.

A woman I met who presented with postcholecystectomy symptoms, particularly those mimicking SOD, found out that her pain all along was a slipped rib. I haven't seen research where a nerve or rib condition could cause nausea, vomiting, diarrhea, etc. unless the nerve and rib are somehow causing an obstruction. That is why I would only consider this diagnosis if your symptom is solely pain.

Cystic stump remnant syndrome: One theory that has been raised in postcholecystectomy support groups and has been theorized by a few doctors is the matter of the cystic duct remnant. Years ago, gallbladders were not removed laparoscopically and were always performed as an open abdominal surgery. I remember when I was 14 years old, my best friend's sister had her gallbladder removed. She had a huge incision that kept her on the couch for over a month.

Back then, most, if not all, of the cystic duct was removed as it was easily done through open surgery. Since the risk of cutting the bile duct or another organ increases if the cystic duct is cut close during laparoscopic surgery, surgeons have opted to leave much of the duct hanging. There is a bundle of nerves connecting the cystic duct with the bile duct and sphincters. If after CCK is released, the body attempts to contract a gallbladder that is no longer there, it may set off the cystic stump and all the nerves associate with it.

Ask your doctor to look at recent scans to see if you have an especially long cystic duct remnant. Unfortunately, most doctors do not think a long cystic duct remnant could cause pain. However, I met a man who had postcholecystectomy pain and got relief by having his cystic duct shortened through surgery.

Histamine Intolerance and Mast Cell Activation Disorder—Histamine is a chemical involved in your immune system, proper digestion, and your central nervous system. Mast cells are produced by the body as an allergic response. Both conditions are a result of either too much histamine build up or mast cell activation. It has been shown that histamine and mast cells play a critical role in liver repair and regeneration and overall intestinal health. Symptoms include rash, hives, diarrhea, headache, nausea/vomiting, itching, abdominal pain, swelling/edema, anxiety, brain fog, fatigue, low blood pressure, and itching.

Although this condition isn't widely linked to postcholecystectomy syndrome, I have met some patients who developed it after their gallbladder was removed. In addition, there was a study of pediatric patients with biliary dyskinesia and gallstones which showed an increase in mast cell density and a moderate to high degree of mast cell activation among these patients.

This condition is difficult to diagnose and treat, but can be identified through food elimination, a tryptase blood test, urine test, endoscopic biopsy, or skin prick test. Staying away from high histamine foods, foods that liberate histamine, and known trigger foods can help. There are also special antihistamines used in severe cases. Some patients report probiotics have helped them.

What You Can Do

Ask your doctor to test for some of these conditions, depending on your symptoms. If they can't, ask to be referred to a physician who has the capability of conducting such tests. If medical doctors have been thorough and you have been through extensive testing, find a good functional medicine practitioner and/or naturopath by searching online, asking friends and family, or your primary care doctor. You may have to interview a few before finding the right one. Ask if they are familiar with the conditions listed previously.

Seek the consult of a good psychiatrist and mental health therapist for your mental health needs. As I've said before, if you didn't have mental health issues prior to getting sick, you now have them thanks to illness, fear of the unknown, and, for some, negative experiences with doctors.

Try acupuncture, hypnotherapy, reiki, yoga, meditating, or any other modality that could realign your digestive system and body energy field. Whatever you can do to de-stress your digestive system, find it. Get your body in balance again!

Re-evaluate the medications you are on and discuss tapering off any with your doctor. If your doctor recommends an antibiotic, ask about an alternative. More digestive issues begin because of antibiotics than anything else I've witnessed.

Be patient. I know this is easier said than done, but time is the best medicine for any condition. Think about it like this. You get a cold and continue to work, burn the candle at both ends, and wonder why after a month you can't get rid of the bronchitis that developed. If everyone stopped what they were doing when they got sick, practiced self-care and natural treatments, and relaxed, I guarantee most wouldn't be ill more than a week. Patience and time are important healers.

Don't give up and don't do this alone. I know how horrible and devastating it is to have unexplained symptoms. I truly do. Stick with people who believe in you and do not doubt your illness, that includes family and friends. Whatever it is that will get you out of the isolation of illness, do it!

My hope is that this book provided you with much-needed answers and information that will result in healing and wellness. Never ever give up hope that you will feel better.

Bibliography
(All Internet citations retrieved June 2017)

Acalovschi M. and Lammert F. The Growing Global Burden of Gallstone Disease. World Gastroenterology Organization. http://www.worldgastroenterology.org/publications/e-wgn/e-wgn-expert-point-of-view-articles-collection/the-growing-global-burden-of-gallstone-disease

Adams,S. (2012, April 27). Why Do So Many Doctors Regret Their Job Choice? http://www.forbes.com/sites/susanadams/2012/04/27/why-do-so-many-doctors-regret-their-job-choice/#616baef07dab

Afamefuna S. and Allen S. Gallbladder Disease. Pathophysiology, Diagnosis, and Treatment Disclosures. *US Pharmacist*. 2013;38(3):33-41.

Chan, H. (2011). Endoscopic Papillary Large Balloon Dilation Alone Without Sphincterotomy for the Treatment of Large Common Bile Duct Stones. BMC Gastroenterology.

Chase, B. Four Bitter Herbs Heal the Liver, Gallbladder, and Other Ailments. Natural News. http://www.naturalnews.com/037460_bitter_herbs_gall_bladder_liver.html#ixzz4XFaokPBk

Choosing Your Digestive Enzymes. Baseline of Health Foundation. https://jonbarron.org/enzymes/enzymes-part-2-3

Duca S., Bãlã O., Al-Hajjar N., Iancu C., Puia I., Munteanu D., and Graur F. Laparoscopic cholecystectomy: incidents and complications. A retrospective analysis of 9542 consecutive laparoscopic operations. *HPB* (Oxford)v.5(3); 2003PMC2020579.

EMDR Humanitarian Assistance Programs, Trauma Recovery Website. http://www.emdrhap.org/content/what-is-emdr/

Fiber: Why It Matters More Than You Think. Experience Life. https://experiencelife.com/article/fiber-why-it-matters-more-than-you-think/

Freeman H. Hepatobiliary and pancreatic disorders in celiac disease." *World Journal of Gastroenterology*. 2006 Mar 14;12(10):1503-8.

Fuentes, A. "Men and Women Are the Same Species!". Psychology Today. https://www.psychologytoday.com/blog/busting-myths-about-human-nature/201205/men-and-women-are-the-same-species

Gallbladder Cancer: Symptoms and Signs. Conquer Cancer Foundation. http://www.cancer.net/cancer-types/gallbladder-cancer/symptoms-and-signs

Gallbladder Disease. Healthline. http://www.healthline.com/health/gallbladder-disease#Overview1

Gallstone Disease: Introduction. Johns Hopkins Hospital. http://www.hopkinsmedicine.org/gastroenterology_hepatology/_pdfs/pancreas_biliary_tract/gallstone_disease.pdf

Gallbladder Disease. Liver Doctor. www.liverdoctor.com

Gallstones: Symptoms and Causes. Mayo Clinic. http://www.mayoclinic.org/diseases-conditions/gallstones/symptoms-causes/dxc-20231395

Gastric Emptying Scan. Healthline. http://www.healthline.com/health/gastric-emptying-scan#uses2

Greer J., Park E., Safren S. (2010 Jan 1). Tailoring Cognitive-Behavioral Therapy to Treat Anxiety Comorbid with Advanced Cancer. Journal of Cognitive Psychotherapy. 24(4): 294–313. Gallbladder. Inner Body. http://www.innerbody.com/image_digeov/dige04-new.html

Hormones, the Pancreas, and Obesity. Discovery's Edge (Mayo Clinic Magazine). November 2010. http://www.mayo.edu/research/discoverys-edge/hormones-pancreas-obesity

How does the Gallbladder Help Digest food? Laparoscopic.md. http://www.laparoscopic.md/digestion/gallbladder

Hurd, K. Gallbladder Disease. Karen Hurd Nutritional Practice. http://www.karenhurd.com/pages/healthtopics/specifichealthconcerns/ht-shc-gallbladderdisease#sthash.OzeuTJJ5.dpuf

Imaging tests to help diagnose digestive problems. WebMD. http://www.webmd.com/digestive-disorders/imaging-tests#1

Jensen, S. and Geibel J. Postcholecystectomy Syndrome. Medscape. http://emedicine.medscape.com/article/192761-overview

Karling P., Norrback K., Adolfsson R., Danielsson A. Gastrointestinal Symptoms are Associated with Hypothalamic-pituitary-adrenal axis Suppression in Healthy Individuals. *Scandinavian Journal of Gastroenterology.* 2007 Nov;42(11):1294-301.

Khan S. Gallbladder Surgery Complications. Buzzle. http://www.buzzle.com/articles/gallbladder-surgery-complications.html

Kline, et al. "Progesterone inhibits gallbladder motility through multiple signaling pathways". Steroids. 2005 Aug;70(9):673-9 http://www.ncbi.nlm.nih.gov/pubmed/15916787

Levine, J. (2015, June 17). The Science of Breathing. Yoga Journal. http://www.yogajournal.com/article/yoga-101/science-breathing

Lingen, J. "The Second Trimester: Constipation, Gas, & Heartburn". Healthline. March 5, 2012.

http://www.healthline.com/health/pregnancy/second-trimester-constipation-gas-heartburn

Luman, W., et al. "Influence of Cholecystectomy on Sphincter of Oddi Motility". Gut. 1997;41:371-374 doi:10.1136/gut.41.3.371. http://gut.bmj.com/content/41/3/371.long

Lv Y., Lau W., Wu H., Chang S., Liu N., Li Y., Deng J. Etiological Causes of Intrahepatic and Extrahepatic Bile Duct Dilatation. *International Journal of New Technology and Research*. ISSN:2454-4116, Volume-1, Issue-8, December 2015 Pages 53-57.

 Mirza, M. (2014, June 25). Ginger Reduces Inflammation and Pain. https://painpatient.com/2014/06/25/ginger-reduces-inflammation-and-pain

Nakauchi L. Beets Detoxify the Liver. Natural News. http://www.naturalnews.com/033025_beets_liver_function.html#ixzz4UuuDn71l

Parkman H., Yates K., Hasler W., Nguyen L., Pasricha P., Snape W., Farrugia G., Koch K., Calles J., Abell T., Sarosiek I., McCallum R., Lee L., Unalp-Arida A., Tonascia J., Hamilton F. Cholecystectomy and Clinical Presentations of Gastroparesis. *Digestive Diseases and Sciences*. 2013 Apr;58(4):1062-73. 2013 Mar 2.

Purcell M. The Health Benefits of Journaling. https://psychcentral.com/lib/the-health-benefits-of-journaling/

Secretion of Bile and the Role of Bile Acids In Digestion. Colorado State University. http://www.vivo.colostate.edu/hbooks/pathphys/digestion/liver/bile.html

Tantia O., Jain M., Khanna S., Sen B. (2008 Jul-Sep). Post cholecystectomy syndrome: Role of cystic duct stump and reintervention by laparoscopic surgery. J Minim Access Surg. 4(3): 71–75.

The Science of Breathing. Yoga Journal.
http://www.yogajournal.com/article/yoga-101/science-breathing/

The Surprising Dangers of CT scans and X-rays. (2015, January 15). Consumer Reports.
http://www.consumerreports.org/cro/magazine/2015/01/the-surprising-dangers-of-ct-sans-and-x-rays/index.htm

Tierney, S., et al. "Estrogen inhibits sphincter of Oddi motility". The Journal of Surgical Research. 1994 Jul;57(1):69-73.

Tierney, S., et al. "Progesterone alters biliary flow dynamics". Annals of Surgery. 1999 Feb; 229(2): 205–209.

Toouli J. Biliary Dyskinesia. *Current Treat Options Gastroenterology*. 2002 Aug;5(4):285-291.

What Are the Functions of Amylase, Protease and Lipase Digestive Enzymes. SFGate.
http://healthyeating.sfgate.com/functions-amylase-protease-lipase-digestive-enzymes-3325.html

Zakko S. and Zakko W. Functional gallbladder disorder in adults. UptoDate. http://www.uptodate.com/contents/functional-gallbladder-disorder-in-adults

Made in the USA
Columbia, SC
20 September 2017